Doppler Color Imaging

CLINICS IN DIAGNOSTIC ULTRASOUND VOLUME 27

Volumes Already Published

Doppler Color Imaging

Edited by

Christopher R.B. Merritt, M.D.

Chairman
Department of Radiology
Ochsner Clinic and the Alton Ochsner Medical Foundation
Clinical Professor
Department of Radiology
Tulane University School of Medicine
New Orleans, Louisiana

Churchill Livingstone
New York, Edinburgh, London, Melbourne, Tokyo

Library of Congress Cataloging-in-Publication Data

Doppler color imaging / edited by Christopher R.B. Merritt.

     p. cm.– (Clinics in diagnostic ultrasound ; v. 27)

    Includes bibliographical references and index.

    ISBN 0-443-08763-6

    1. Doppler ultrasonography. I. Merritt, Christopher R.B., date
    II. Series.

    [DNLM: 1. Echocardiography, Doppler. W1 CL831BC v.27 / WG
  141.5.E2 D6915]

  RC78.7.U4D65 1992

  616.07'543–dc20

  DNLM/DLC

  for Library of Congress   92-6918
                                                     CIP

Distributed in the United Kingdom by Churchill Livingstone, Robert Stevenson House, 1–3 Baxter's Place, Leith Walk, Edinburgh EH1 3AF, and by associated companies, branches, and representatives throughout the world.

Accurate indications, adverse reactions, and dosage schedules for drugs are provided in this book, but it is possible that they may change. The reader is urged to review the package information data of the manufacturers of the medications mentioned.

The Publishers have made every effort to trace the copyright holders for borrowed material. If they have inadvertently overlooked any, they will be pleased to make the necessary arrangements at the first opportunity.

Acquisitions Editor: *Nancy Mullins*
Copy Editor: *Bridgett Dickinson*
Production Designer: *Patricia McFadden*
Production Supervisor: *Jeanine Furino*

Printed in Singapore

First published in 1992   7 6 5 4 3 2 1

Contributors

Edward I. Bluth, M.D.

Associate Head, Section of Ultrasound, Department of Radiology, Ochsner Clinic and the Alton Ochsner Medical Foundation; Clinical Professor, Department of Radiology, Tulane University School of Medicine, New Orleans, Louisiana

Gregory P. Borkowski, M.D.

Chairman of Hospital Radiology, Department of Radiology, Cleveland Clinic Foundation, Cleveland , Ohio

Cara Case, R.D.M.S.

Research Associate, Department of Diagnostic Radiology, Yale University School of Medicine, New Haven, Connecticut

Lynwood Hammers, D.O.

Associate Professor, Department of Diagnostic Radiology, Yale University School of Medicine; Director, Ultrasound Section, Department of Diagnostic Radiology, Yale-New Haven Hospital, New Haven, Connecticut

Frederick W. Kremkau, Ph.D.

Professor and Director, Center for Medical Ultrasound, Bowman Gray School of Medicine of Wake Forest University, Winston-Salem, North Carolina

Christopher R.B. Merritt, M.D.

Chairman, Department of Radiology, Ochsner Clinic and the Alton Ochsner Medical Foundation; Clinical Professor, Department of Radiology, Tulane University School of Medicine, New Orleans, Louisiana

David M. Paushter, M.D.

Head, Section of Abdominal Imaging, Department of Radiology, Cleveland Clinic Foundation, Cleveland, Ohio

John S. Pellerito, M.D.

Assistant Professor, Department of Diagnostic Radiology, Yale University School of Medicine, New Haven, Connecticut

Kenneth J.W. Taylor, M.D., Ph.D., F.A.C.P.
Professor and Academic Director, Department of Diagnostic Radiology, Yale University School of Medicine, New Haven, Connecticut

Preface

At the American Institute of Ultrasound in Medicine meeting in the fall of 1983, I received my first glimpse of what was to become Doppler color imaging. As we sat in the lounge of the New York Hilton, Mr. David Croniser, representing a group later to be known as Quantum Medical Systems, sketched out an idea for a new type of ultrasound device. The proposed instrument would be capable of imaging both tissue and blood flow simultaneously from vessels throughout the body. The challenges to be overcome in making such a device were formidable. The detection of low signal objects moving in areas of high clutter and noise would require use of new technology, much of it derived from defense applications. As we talked, Dave produced rough images of what the final output of such a device might look like–blood vessels showing flow in bright shades of red and blue. I was hooked on the concept and over the next year received updates on the progress being made in converting these ideas into a clinical device. At the meeting of the Radiological Society of North America in December of 1984, I was shown the first images, which had been produced only days before by an engineering prototype. These images, although crude by current standards, showed unequivocally the possibility that a clinically useful device might be produced.

Six months later, in the summer of 1985, a huge and ugly box with open circuit boards and a maze of exposed wiring arrived at our laboratory. This was the company's first clinical prototype Doppler color scanner, and we had agreed to perform its initial clinical testing. Applying the instrument to a series of patients in an investigational protocol, we saw for the first time features of blood flow within living patients that had never been imaged before. Our preliminary observations were first presented at the meeting of the Society of Radiologists in Ultrasound in October of 1985. There was a mixed reaction from the members in attendance. Some agreed immediately that Doppler color imaging was a major advance in ultrasound technology, while others considered it novel, but questioned its potential as a clinical tool. Now, 6 years later, there can be no question that Doppler color imaging has assumed a critically important role, which extends into all areas of ultrasonography. This book, which presents the experience of some of the researchers who have led the way in exploring the application of color flow imaging to a variety of problems, provides a timely and comprehensive update on the role of Doppler color imaging in ultrasound.

Christopher R.B. Merritt, M.D.

Contents

1

Introduction

Christopher R. B. Merritt

Ultrasound is the most rapidly growing of all imaging modalities. This growth results from the acceptance by clinicians of the clinical value of ultrasound in an ever-increasing range of important new applications. Among the recent and most important new applications of ultrasonography is Doppler color imaging (DCI). By combining high-resolution tissue imaging with the simultaneous display of flow information as well as conventional Doppler spectral analysis, DCI has, for the first time, provided the opportunity for detailed noninvasive assessment not only of morphology but also of function as reflected in organ blood supply and perfusion. Since its clinical introduction in the mid-1980s, DCI has become widely accepted as a means of evaluating the peripheral vascular system and as an adjunct to gray-scale imaging for numerous uses in the abdomen, pelvis, pregnant uterus, and extremities. The important applications for which DCI has become a useful, and in some cases essential, adjunct to conventional ultrasound imaging and duplex Doppler will be covered in detail in the following chapters.

The development of DCI technology is the most recent step in a series of technological advances marking the evolution of diagnostic ultrasound instrumentation since its simple beginnings in the 1950s. In reaching its current level of clinical utility, ultrasound has undergone several critical transformations over the past 40 years, each with major clinical impact. The possibility of using ultrasound for medical diagnosis was initially explored in the early 1950s by using A-mode display. Although crude by current standards, these efforts were of great importance because they indicated the possibility of obtaining unique and clinically useful information by using acoustic energy. In the early 1960s the development of bistable B-mode display opened the door to two-dimensional imaging of the body. Although these bistable instruments were limited in their widespread clinical use, they and the pioneers who explored their diagnostic potential laid the groundwork for the ultrasound imaging revolution of the 1970s that was brought about by the development of gray-scale scan converters. With these devices, readily recognizable images of the parenchyma of major organs, rather than simply their outline, were produced. By the mid-1970s ultrasound was well on its way to becoming an established and acceptable diagnostic imaging procedure. In the late 1970s the commercial introduction of real-time imaging, duplex Doppler, and new transducer technology greatly extended the range of clinical applications of ultrasound as well as its clinical acceptance. Each of the advances in technology and hardware that has characterized the evolution of diagnostic ultrasound has resulted in major improvements in the efficacy of ultrasound as a primary imaging method and has permitted ultrasound to enjoy continued growth despite revolutionary developments in other imaging modalities, such as computed tomography (CT) and magnetic resonance imaging (MRI).

The most recent in the series of major technological achievements in diagnostic ultrasonography is related to the revolution in computer technology of the 1980s. To generate a single Doppler color image it is necessary to collect and process an immense amount of data from the backscattered ultrasound. This requires an enormous amount of computing power and sophisticated, highly efficient software. Before the availability of affordable high-speed computer processing, it was not feasible to simultaneously process both tissue and flow data from the backscattered ultrasound signal and generate an image of blood flow in real time. Now, with current computer power, a number of commercially available instruments that allow real-time simultaneous display of color-encoded flow along with high-resolution tissue detail have been developed.

Real-time color-flow mapping devices were first developed and used for cardiac applications.[1-7] This cardiac instrumentation has been described in the literature by a variety of terms, including *color-coded Doppler, Doppler angiography, 2-D* (two-dimensional) *Doppler, Doppler color flow mapping, Doppler color flow imaging* (DCFI), *color Doppler flow imaging* (CDFI), *color Doppler imaging* (CDI), *Doppler color imaging* (DCI), and *angiodynography.*[8] These terms tend to be somewhat confusing because new methods developed to allow the simultaneous imaging of tissue and flow are not really distinguished from earlier, less sophisticated techniques. For example, Doppler color flow mapping has been used to describe both a frequency mapping system, which does not employ real-time, and a cardiac phased-array real-time imager.[1,9] Although arguments can be made to support several of these terms, the terms most widely used include *Doppler color imaging, color Doppler imaging,* and *Doppler color flow imaging.* Each of these terms accurately indicates the fundamental elements of the technology—namely the use of Doppler to obtain flow-related data, the display of this information in color, and the use of an imaging format for data display. Since the image provided by most currently available systems is based on data derived from analysis of the Doppler-shifted frequency spectrum rather than a direct assessment of flow, the terms *Doppler color imaging* and *color Doppler imaging* are more appropriate than the term *Doppler color flow imaging* we originally proposed.[8] This is particularly true when one considers the useful information provided by these instruments in demonstrating conditions not related to flow, such as the tissue motion accompanying bruits. For this book we have elected to use the term *Doppler color imaging* or its acronym DCI to describe the techniques and instrumentation currently in general use.

Over the past 40 years or so, there has been a tendency for new technology to appear in the medical marketplace without the prior definition of a clear clinical role for it. In many cases the medical profession has been asked to evaluate a new technology to see whether it has a medical use, rather than to identify a specific clinical need and then search for the technology best suited to fill it. By contrast, the development of DCI technology was stimulated by a clear and important clinical need. The determination of vessel patency, the presence and direction of blood flow, and the evaluation of organ perfusion have been goals of diagnostic imaging since the turn of the century. This need has been addressed, with various degrees of success, by angiography, dynamic CT, radionuclide flow imaging, MRI, and Doppler ultrasonography.

Duplex and continuous-wave Doppler ultrasound have been used clinically for more than 20 years and have been the mainstay of the noninvasive assessment of blood flow. Despite its proven utility, Doppler spectral analysis has evolved relatively slowly compared with the rapid strides in other applications of diagnostic ultrasound. Although duplex Doppler scanners combine B-mode and Doppler for both tissue imaging and flow measurement, the use of duplex Doppler ultrasound has been restricted to a relatively few well-defined indications in cardiac diagnosis, in the evaluation of carotid and peripheral vascular disease, and more recently

in obstetrics and abdominal diagnosis.[10] A major limitation of duplex Doppler ultrasound is that flow information is obtained only from a highly restricted sample volume and not from the remainder of the image (Fig. 1-1). To obtain maximum information with duplex Doppler ultrasound, a skilled operator must perform careful sampling of all of the sites within the vessel lumen where flow disturbances are likely to be found. A preferable approach would be a method allowing evaluation of flow characteristics throughout the entire image combined with high-resolution display of the vessel wall and surrounding tissue features. This approach is exactly what is provided by combining Doppler flow and tissue imaging in DCI (Fig. 1-2). With DCI, all of the features and benefits of spectral Doppler sampling are retained and the unique new capability of global Doppler sampling—the ability to obtain flow-related information from throughout an area of interest—is added. In our

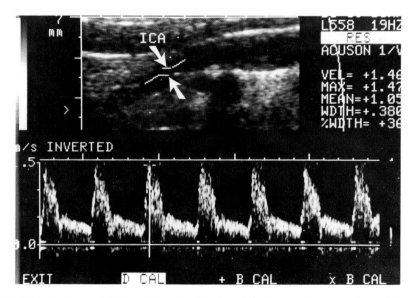

Fig. 1-1 Limitations of duplex Doppler. Duplex Doppler permits sampling of flow data from only the area contained within the Doppler sample volume (arrows). The Doppler waveform provides a graphic display of the Doppler-shifted frequencies as they vary with time.

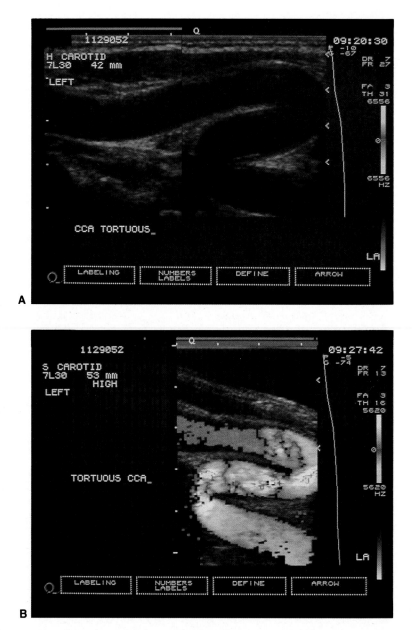

Fig. 1-2 Doppler color imaging. With DCI, flow is sampled from throughout the image and, when present, is displayed in color along with gray-scale information from tissue. **(A)** Gray-scale image of a tortuous common carotid artery. **(B)** Flow within the vessel is shown by using DCI. The global sampling and display of flow information possible with DCI represents its major advantage over duplex Doppler.

view, DCI does not replace duplex Doppler but expands its range of applications and usefulness.

Working in a complementary rather than a competitive fashion, duplex ultrasound and DCI now serve as valuable adjuncts to imaging in several ways. Vessels may be quickly and positively identified and reliably differentiated from nonvascular structures. With Doppler it is possible to determine the net direction of blood flow as well as brief changes in flow direction that may occur during the course of the cardiac cycle. Doppler permits the identification of vessel occlusion and may be used to infer the presence and degree of vessel narrowing. Finally, Doppler aids in the characterization of flow to organs, transplants, tumors, and the fetus. Although most of the work with Doppler ultrasound has emphasized the detection of occlusion, stenosis, and flow disturbances in major vessels, the importance of Doppler information in the inference of abnormalities in the peripheral vascular bed of an organ or tissue deserves special emphasis. Changes in the spectral waveform, or, in the case of DCI, in the appearance of flow in diastole,

provide insight into the resistance of the vascular bed supplied by the vessel and, although not specific, may indicate changes due to a variety of disorders (Fig. 1-3). The specific changes accompanying these abnormalities are discussed in detail in the following chapters.

A growing interest in the use of Doppler for abdominal, pelvic, obstetric, and oncologic applications, as well as in evaluation of the carotid and peripheral vascular systems, makes this review of DCI especially timely. Our experience in the performance of approximately 20,000 DCI examinations since scanning our first patient with a prototype instrument in 1985 has confirmed our initial impression of the clinical potential of this new approach to ultrasound imaging. In our practice, DCI complemented by image-guided pulsed Doppler spectral analysis has largely replaced simple duplex Doppler in carotid, peripheral arterial, and venous applications. Although it is difficult to prove that increased diagnostic accuracy has been added by DCI in these examinations, we have no doubt that the use of DCI has resulted in greater diagnostic information, shorter ex-

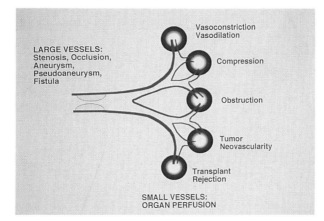

Fig. 1-3 Importance of flow information. DCI aids in the inference of changes in blood flow and organ perfusion at multiple levels. In large arteries and veins, stenosis and occlusion may be detected and measured. In small peripheral vessels, changes in resistance related to a variety of diseases may be detected. The ability of Doppler ultrasound to provide clinically useful information throughout the circulatory system is one of its most important features.

amination time, and higher levels of confidence in both normal and abnormal diagnoses. In the evaluation of vessels in the abdomen, pelvis, and fetus, DCI has resulted in similar benefits and made unequivocal contributions to the care of many patients.

REFERENCES

1. Switzer DF, Nanda NC: Doppler color flow mapping. Ultrasound Med Biol 11:403, 1985
2. Bommer WJ, Miller L: Real-time two-dimensional color-flow Doppler: enhanced Doppler flow imaging in the diagnosis of cardiovascular disease, abstracted. Am J Cardiol 49:944, 1982
3. Namekawa K, Kasai C, Tsukamoto M, et al: Imaging of blood flow using autocorrelation. Ultrasound Med Biol 8:138, 1982
4. Suzuki Y, Kambara H, Kadota K, et al: Detection of intracardiac shunt flow in atrial septal defect using a real-time two-dimensional color-coded Doppler flow imaging system and comparison with contrast two-dimensional echocardiography. Am J Cardiol 56:347, 1985
5. Miyatake K, Okamoto M, Kinoshita N, et al: Clinical applications of a new type of real-time two-dimensional Doppler flow imaging system. Am J Cardiol 54:857, 1984
6. Ortiz E, Robinson PJ, Deanfield JE, et al: Localisation of ventricular septal defects by simultaneous display of superimposed colour Doppler and cross sectional echocardiographic images. Br Heart J 54:53, 1985
7. Dagli SV, Nanda NC, Roitman D, et al: Evaluation of aortic dissection by Doppler color flow mapping. Am J Cardiol 56:497, 1985
8. Merritt CRB: Doppler color flow imaging. J Clin Ultrasound 15:591, 1987
9. Ackroyd N, Lane R, Dart L, et al: Colour-coded carotid Doppler imaging: an angiographic comparison of 324 bifurcations. Aust NZ J Surg 54:509, 1984
10. Taylor KJW, Burns PN: Duplex Doppler scanning in the pelvis and abdomen. Ultrasound Med Biol 11:643, 1985

2

Principles and Instrumentation

Frederick W. Kremkau

Doppler color imaging (DCI) is a technique in which two-dimensional real-time presentations of blood flow information are displayed for medical diagnostic purposes. The colors are given hues, saturations, and brightnesses to indicate presence, direction, speed, and type (laminar, disturbed, turbulent) of flow. This information is superimposed on the two-dimensional gray-scale anatomic cross-sectional sonographic image. As with conventional sonography, an ultrasonic transducer is placed on the surface of the patient, with acoustic contact ensured by use of coupling gel.[1] Pulses of ultrasound are sent into the patient, and returning echoes are processed to present the color-flow information on the display. The color-flow presentation provides information regarding the presence, qualitative direction (toward or away from the transducer), speed, and type (normal or abnormal) of flow.

PRINCIPLES OF COLOR FLOW

In color-flow imaging, a pulse-echo technique is used. In most cases, the Doppler effect is utilized.[2] This requires that pulses be longer (more cycles) than those used for gray-scale anatomic imaging (Fig. 2-1). However, the two techniques are quite similar. As the pulse of ultrasound travels through tissues, echoes are generated that are received by the transducer in sequence from nearest to deepest. These are presented along a scan line on the display representing the travel path from the transducer in the appropriate direction into the patient's tissues (Fig. 2-2A). Non-Doppler-shifted echo amplitude is presented as brightness (gray-scale) in its proper location along the scan line.[1] For Doppler-shifted echoes, the Doppler shift is determined for each echo and presented as color at the appropriate location (Fig. 2-2B). Color indicates primarily the qualitative direction of flow but can also indicate the speed and character of flow. Unlike gray-scale anatomic imaging, several pulses are needed to determine Doppler shifts and to generate a single-color scan line (Fig. 2-1). The process is repeated, sending pulses through the entire tissue cross-section to be interrogated in linear or sector scan format, filling the memory with Doppler-shifted echo information in lo-

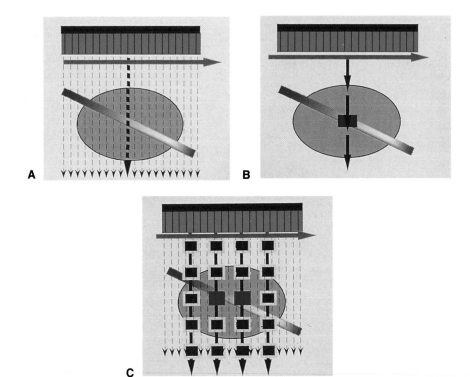

Fig. 2-1 Operating modes. **(A)** In scanned operating modes, short pulses of ultrasound are emitted in a series of sequential scan lines to generate the real-time image (dashed arrows). Any given point in the image is exposed only briefly (dark arrow). **(B)** In pulsed-Doppler operating modes, a series of relatively long pulses is transmitted along a path that may be steered by the user. Echoes from targets in the sample volume (red box) are processed for Doppler frequency shift data. **(C)** In color-Doppler operating modes, more pulses are used for each scan line than for imaging alone and both tissue (blue boxes) and flow data (red boxes) are sampled from along each line.

cations corresponding to its origin in the tissues and then displaying in corresponding locations on the instrument display. Commonly, in each location on the display either gray-scale or color-flow information is presented, but not both. The result is a two-dimensional display with gray-scale representation of cross-sectional anatomy and flow information superimposed in color at appropriate locations and presented in various hues, saturations, and brightnesses (Fig. 2-3).

DOPPLER EFFECT

The Doppler effect is a change in wavelength or frequency of sound resulting from motion of a sound source, receiver, or reflector.[2] The Doppler effect applies generally to any kind of wave, but in this discussion only waves of ultrasound are considered. In medical diagnostic applications in which ultrasound is used, the source and receiver of the ultrasound is the transducer, which is stationary. An exception to this is mechanical

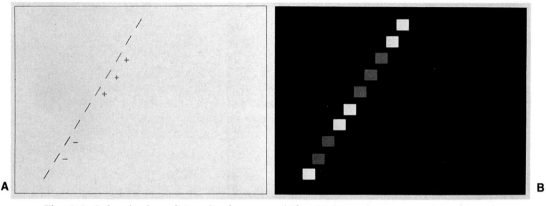

Fig. 2-2 Color display of Doppler frequency shift. **(A)** Ten echoes are received as a pulse travels through tissues. Three (red) have positive Doppler shifts, and two (blue) have negative shifts. **(B)** The echoes are shown as red and blue pixels, respectively, on the color-flow display. (From Kremkau,[2] with permission.)

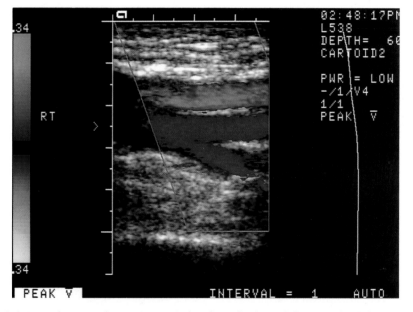

Fig. 2-3 Vascular Doppler imaging. Color-flow display of the superficial femoral artery (red) and the superficial and deep femoral veins (blue) by using a linear-array transducer. The gray-scale anatomic image is composed of vertical parallel scan lines. By phasing, the color scan lines are angled 20 degrees away from vertical. Blue and red indicate positive and negative Doppler shifts, respectively. The vessel nearest the transducer (top) is filled with echoes having negative Doppler shifts, indicating flow from left to right. The two lower vessels that merge into one are filled with positive Doppler shifts, indicating flow from right to left.

transducers (including annular arrays). However, they do not move while acquiring Doppler data. Their motion would not produce a Doppler shift in any case because it is perpendicular to the sound propagation direction. The motion, then, that produces the Doppler effect is that of the moving blood. Cells (primarily erythrocytes) in the flowing blood produce the Doppler-shifted echoes that are received by the transducer, allowing color-flow presentation on the display. The change in frequency between the ultrasound pulses emitted and those received depends on the speed of blood flow, its direction relative to the sound beam direction, the frequency of the emitted ultrasound, and the speed of sound. The Doppler equation relates these quantities and shows the dependence of Doppler shift on them. Doppler shift, f_D, is the difference between transmitted and received frequencies:

$$f_D = \frac{2f_0\, v \cdot \cos\theta}{c}$$

where f_0 is the frequency of transmitted ultrasound, v is the speed of blood flow, θ is the Doppler angle (discussed below), and c is the speed of sound. The faster the blood flows toward or away from the transducer, the greater the Doppler shift will be. For a given blood flow, the higher the operating frequency the greater the Doppler shift. For a given operating frequency and blood flow velocity (speed and direction), the Doppler shift will increase as the ultrasound propagation direction becomes more parallel to the flow direction. As the angle θ (the Doppler angle) between these two directions increases, the Doppler shift decreases and approaches zero at a perpendicular Doppler angle (Fig. 2-4). Doppler color-flow displays thus have an angle dependence like that of other Doppler techniques. Some instruments calibrate their display of color information in terms of flow speed (in meters per second or centimeters per second), incorporating the operating frequency and sound speed into the Doppler equation. In this calibration, the Doppler angle is commonly assumed to be zero (Figs. 2-5A and B), but this is generally incorrect. In some cases angle correction allows proper calibration of color presentation (Fig. 2-5C). The Doppler shift information presented in color on the display is, then, a result of flow speed, flow direction, ultrasound propagation direction, and emitted frequency.

TRANSDUCERS

Various types of transducers are used in color-flow imaging. They include linear, convex, phased, and annular arrays. The operating principles of these various arrays are discussed elsewhere.[1,3] The linear array produces a rectangular image in which gray-scale scan lines are usually vertical (Figs. 2-3 and 2-4) but may be at some other angle (Fig. 2-6). The color-flow information may cover the entire field of view (Fig. 2-4) or may be limited to a box within the gray-scale field with a shape that is either a rectangle (Fig. 2-7A), a parallelogram (Figs. 2-7B and C), or a sector area (Fig. 2-8A and B). The parallelogram shape is generated by sending pulses for color at some angle away from the perpendicular (e.g., 20 degrees) by phasing. Angled box placement at depth is sometimes limited (Figs. 2-7D and E). The sector area is generated by sector transducers (convex, phased, and annular arrays). The color information can be provided throughout the entire display. If phased steering is not used, it may be necessary to introduce an acoustically transparent wedge between the transducer elements and the skin to avoid a Doppler angle of near 90 degrees (Fig. 2-5C). The convex array produces a sector image (Fig. 2-8A). Phasing is not used in the convex array for steering. Phasing is commonly used with linear and convex arrays for focusing. Figures 2-3, 2-7A, and 2-8A are focused by phasing at depths of 2.5, 4.5, and 2.0 cm,

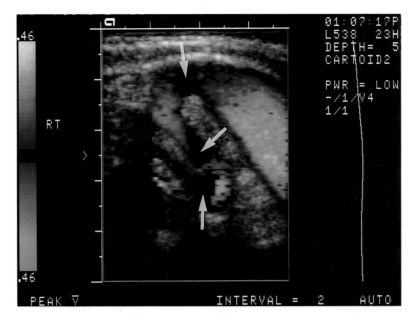

Fig. 2-4 Doppler angle effects. In this image of a tortuous vessel, various Doppler angles are involved. The two red regions indicate positive Doppler shifts with flow toward the transducer. The two blue regions indicate negative Doppler shifts with flow away from the transducer. The uncolored regions within the vessel (arrows) indicate no Doppler shifts. This is because the flow is perpendicular to the color scan lines in these regions (90-degree Doppler angle), yielding zero Doppler shift. It is important to realize that lack of Doppler shift does not necessarily mean no flow.

respectively. Phased arrays produce sector images by steering the beam from one edge of the display to the other by phasing. Focusing is also accomplished by phasing (Figs. 2-8B and C). Annular-phased arrays are two-dimensionally focused by phasing but must be scanned mechanically. Normally, this means that they cannot be used for color imaging, because each color scan line requires that several pulses be sent out along the same path. With mechanical scanning the transducer moves between subsequent pulses and does not send out each pulse in the group (ensemble) along the same path. However, transducers that use digitally driven stepping motors instead of conventionally driven motors can be operated in such a way that they remain stationary while a group of pulses is sent out a given path and then rapidly trans-

late to the next direction for the next group of pulses. With this kind of driving mechanism, mechanically driven transducers (and thus annular-phased arrays) may be used in color-flow imaging (Fig. 2-8D).

PRINCIPLES OF COLOR DISPLAY

Every color has three basic components in its presentation: hue, saturation, and luminance (brightness). Hue is the color observed (red, green, blue, etc); saturation is the concentration of the color (pale, deep, etc); brightness is amount of light (dark, bright, etc) in the presented color. Hue is our subjective interpretation (gradation of color) of the frequency of the light we see (Fig. 2-9).

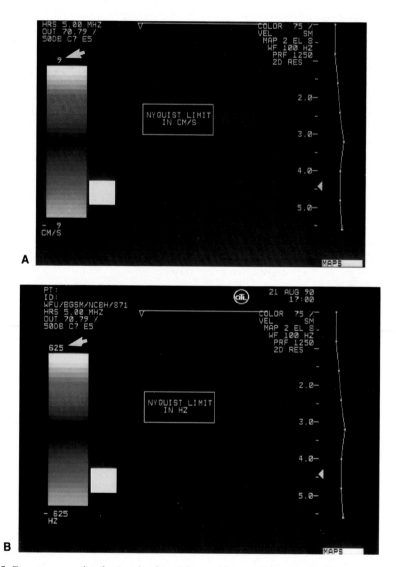

Fig. 2-5 Frequency and velocity display. The maximum flow speed **(A)** in cm/s and the corresponding Doppler shift **(B)** in Hz are indicated by the arrows in the two displays. Substituting the flow speed (9 cm/s), the Doppler shift frequency (625 Hz), the operating frequency (5 MHz), and the sound speed (1,540 m/s) into the Doppler equation yields a value for the cosine of the Doppler angle equal to unity. Since the cosine of an angle of 0 degrees is unity, it is apparent that this instrument is assuming a Doppler angle of 0 degrees in the calibration of the color presentation. This assumption is correct only when the flow is parallel to the color scan lines. (*Figure continues.*)

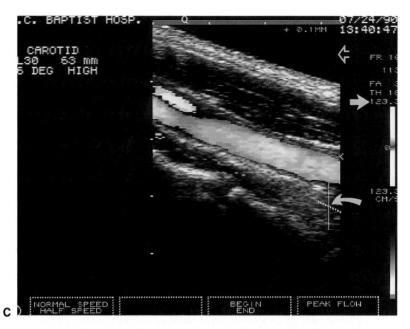

Fig. 2-5 (*Continued*). **(C)** Color scan from a linear array in which the vessel is not parallel to the array face because of a wedge (open arrow). This provides a nonperpendicular Doppler angle for vessels parallel to the skin. Angle correction is provided by the operator in this scan (curved arrow) so that the color calibration to display velocity (arrow) is correct.

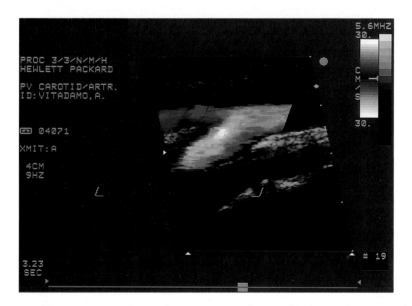

Fig. 2-6 Different image and Doppler scanning angles. In this image the gray-scale scan lines are angled 13 degrees to the right of vertical while the color scan lines are angled 20 degrees to the left of vertical.

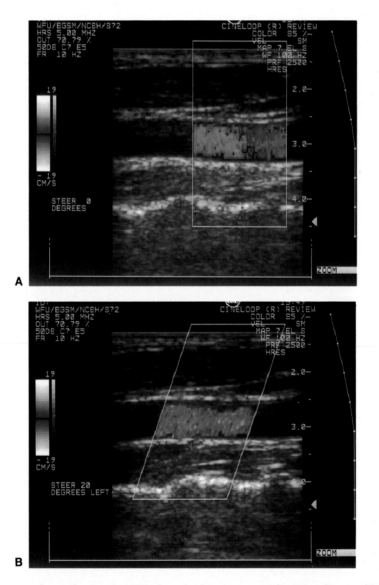

Fig. 2-7 Doppler angle steering. **(A)** The color box is a rectangle with color scan lines parallel to the gray-scale lines. The color reversal in the vessel is due to a slight upward concavity, resulting in slightly negative Doppler shifts on the right and slightly positive Doppler shifts on the left. **(B)** The color box is steered 20 degrees to the left so that color scan lines are not parallel to gray-scale scan lines. The flow is from right to left in the vessel, yielding negative Doppler shifts (blue). **(C)** The color box is steered 20 degrees to the right, yielding positive Doppler shifts in the vessel. **(D)** The color box placed between 4 and 5 cm in depth cannot be translated to the left past its present position. This is because the angled scan line for the left edge of the box has come from the left end of the linear-array transducer **(E)**. (From Kremkau,[4] with permission.) (*Figure continues.*)

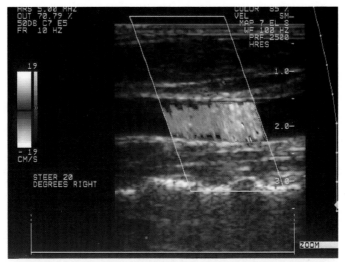

C

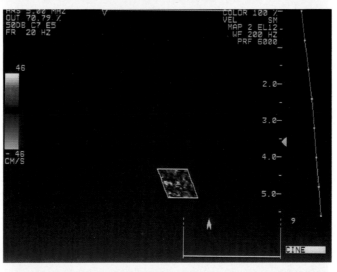

D

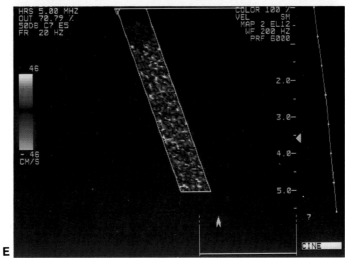

E

Fig. 2-7 (*Continued*).

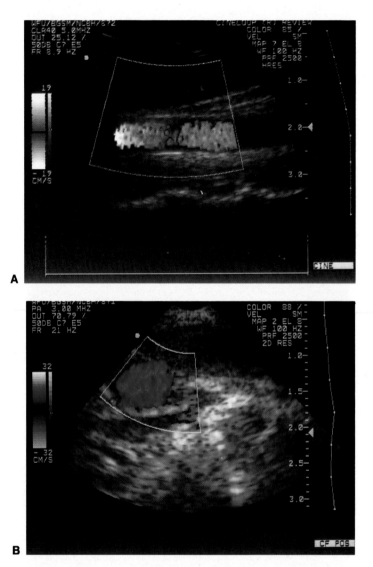

Fig. 2-8 Arrays. **(A)** Display produced by a convex linear-array transducer. The color change results from the changing scan-line angles with respect to the flow proceeding from the right side, where they are experiencing approaching flow, to the left side, where they are experiencing receding flow. **(B)** Scan produced by a phased array with the color box steered to the left portion of the gray-scale scan. (*Figure continues.*)

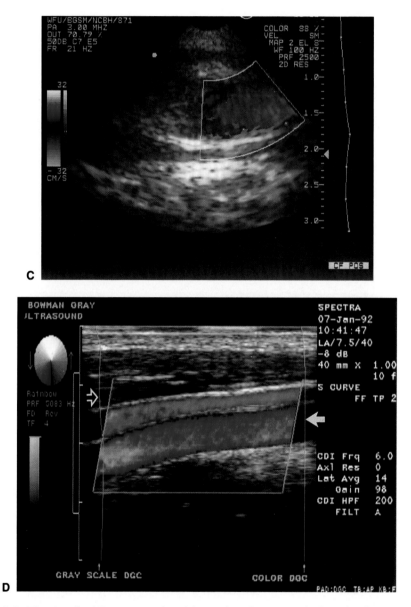

Fig. 2-8 (*Continued*). (**C**) Scan produced by a phased array with the color box steered to the right portion of the gray-scale scan. (**D**) Display of gray-scale and color flow with an annular-array transducer. In this display, a TGC curve (solid arrow) applied to the color presentation is shown. The TGC curve for the gray-scale image (open arrow) is on the left.

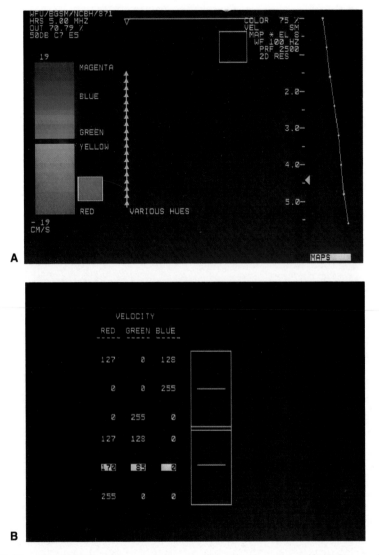

Fig. 2-9 Hue. **(A)** Various hues are shown on this color bar, proceeding from red through orange, yellow, green, and blue to magenta. They are all presented with equal brightness. **(B)** The contributions of red, green, and blue at six different locations of the bar are shown quantitatively in the three columns. For example, at the bottom of the bar, maximum red (255) is the only color present. Nearly halfway up the bar, equal contributions of red and green (127 and 128) are present, yielding yellow. Two-thirds red and one-third green yields orange; and equal amounts of red and blue yield magenta at the top. (*Figure continues.*)

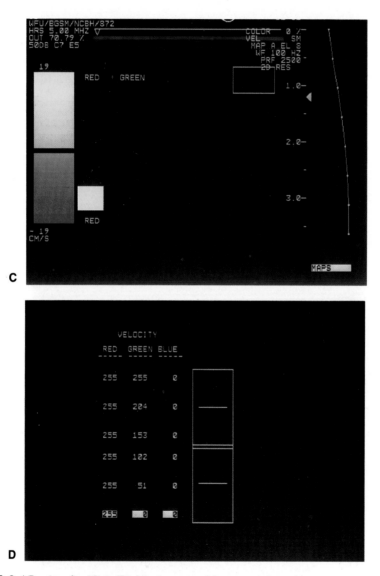

Fig. 2-9 (*Continued*). **(C & D)** Maximum red is present from bottom to top, while green increases from zero to maximum yielding yellow at the top. (*Figure continues.*)

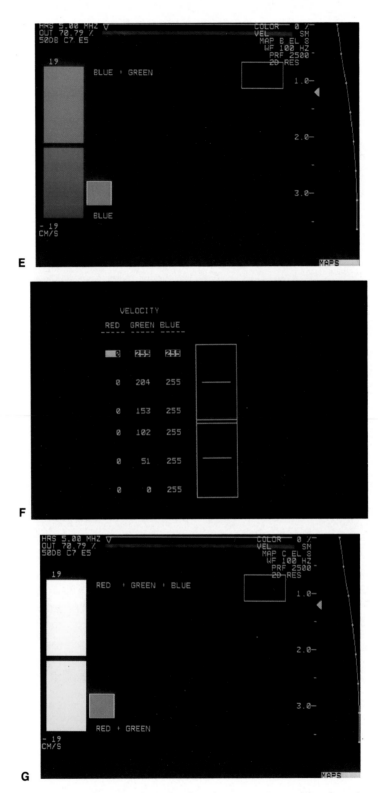

Fig. 2-9 (*Continued*). **(E & F)** The color bar shows maximum blue from bottom to top, while green increases from zero to maximum, yielding cyan at the top. **(G & H)** In this color bar, maximum red and maximum green are present throughout, while blue increases from zero at the bottom to maximum at the top, yielding white. (*Figure continues.*)

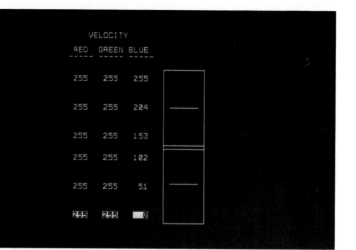

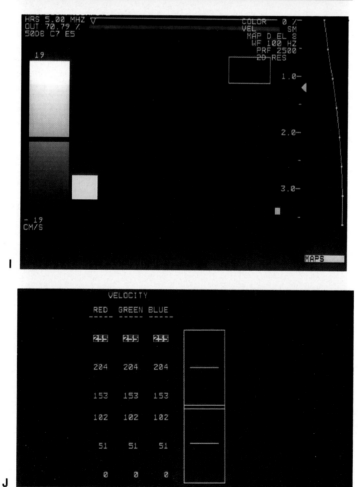

Fig. 2-9 (*Continued*). **(I & J)** Equal amounts of red, green, and blue are present throughout this color bar, with values increasing from zero at the bottom to maximum (255) at the top. This yields a gray bar proceeding from black through increasing brightnesses to white. (From Kremkau,[4] with permission.)

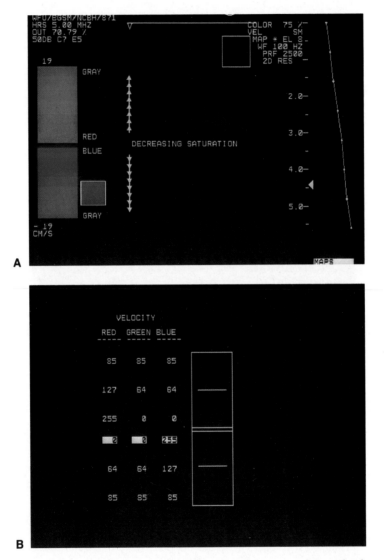

Fig. 2-10 Saturation and brightness. **(A & B)** From the center of the color bar to the top and bottom extremes, red and blue saturation decrease to gray (equal values of red, green, and blue) with constant brightness. (*Figure continues.*)

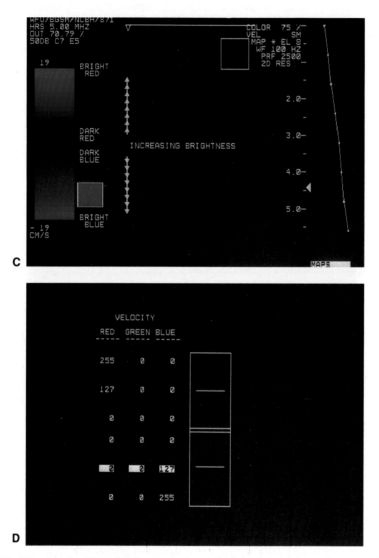

Fig. 2-10 (*Continued*). **(C & D)** From the center of the color bar to the top and bottom extremes, red and blue increase in brightness. (*Figure continues.*)

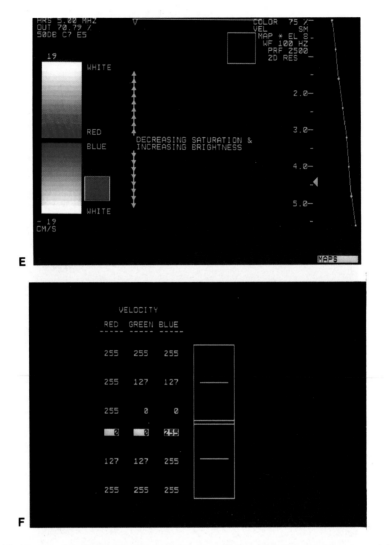

Fig. 2-10 (*Continued*). **(E & F)** From the center of the color bar to the top and bottom extremes, red and blue simultaneously decrease in saturation and increase in brightness, progressing from dark, deep colors to bright white (maximum red, green, and blue).

We even associate colors with various moods and feelings ("seeing red," "being green with envy," and "feeling blue on Monday"). Light is an electromagnetic wave of extremely high frequency (approximately 500 × 10⁶ MHz) that is detected by the eyes and sensed by the brain. The lowest-frequency light humans can see is perceived as red (below that is the invisible infrared). Increasing frequency takes us through orange, yellow, green, blue, and violet light, which is the highest-frequency light we can see (beyond that is the invisible ultraviolet). The retina contains three types of color-sensitive cells (cones), which respond primarily to red, green, and blue frequencies. These colors are called *primary colors* because when they are mixed, nearly any other color can be produced (Fig. 2-9). Equal amounts red and green yield yellow (Figs. 2-9C and D), blue and green yield cyan (Figs. 2-9E and F), and red and blue yield magenta (Figs. 2-9A and

B [top]). Equal amounts of red, green, and blue yield white (Figs. 2-9G to J). Saturation (also called chroma) is the concentration of the hue mixed with white (Fig. 2-10). Low saturation presents a pale color (i.e., washed out with white). High saturation indicates that little white has been added, yielding a deep, or strong, hue. Brightness (also called luminance, luminosity, intensity, or value) is the amount of light emitted per unit area (Fig. 2-10). A low value yields a dark presentation, whereas a high value yields a bright presentation. Figures 2-10E and F show the result of the combination of decreasing saturation and increasing brightness.

DOPPLER INSTRUMENTS

Continuous-wave (CW) and pulsed-duplex Doppler instruments present Doppler flow information from one sample volume. For CW instruments, this sample volume is rather large, consisting of the overlapping region of the transmit and receive transducer element beams.[2] In pulsed-duplex instruments, the sample volume is adjustable and can be quite small (1 or 2 mm in each dimension). In both types of instruments, the Doppler information is presented audibly and as a spectral display (i.e., a plot of Doppler shift versus time).[2] In color-flow instruments, Doppler information is acquired from many locations within the color region (color box or color window). This information is presented two-dimensionally from all these locations and changes with time. A block diagram of a color-flow instrument is given in Figure 2-11. The instrument consists of a pulser that includes beam formation and steering functions, a receiver that performs both conventional gray-scale amplitude detection functions and Doppler detection functions, a memory, and a display.[1] In some instruments the receiver is unified (syn-

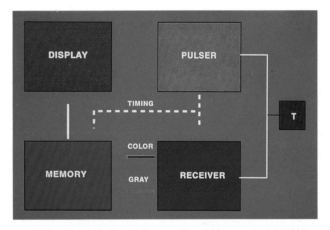

Fig. 2-11 Block diagram of a DCI instrument. The pulser produces electric pulses that drive the transducer (T). It also produces timing pulses that, through the dashed path, tell the receiver and memory when the transducer has been driven. The transducer (acting as a source) produces an ultrasound pulse for each electric pulse applied. For each echo received from the tissues, an electric voltage is produced by the transducer (acting as a receiving transducer). These voltages go to the receiver, where they are processed to a form suitable for storing in memory. The receiver demodulates the non-Doppler-shifted echoes, retaining their amplitude, which is sent to the memory via the "gray" path. The Doppler shifts of Doppler-shifted echoes are determined by the receiver and delivered to the memory via the "color" path. Electric information from memory drives the display, which produces a visual image of the cross-sectional anatomy and flow acquired by the system.

chronous), whereas in others it is a dual receiver (asynchronous), with the gray-scale and Doppler functions carried out independently. Gray-scale and Doppler information is stored in the memory in appropriate locations and presented on the display for viewing. Clearly, a color television monitor is required in these instruments. The high rate of echo return and presentation on the display does not permit determination of the Doppler spectrum for all the Doppler samples along each color scan line using the Fourier transform technique, as is done with spectral displays for one sample volume. In addition, there is no convenient way to present this two-dimensional information (Doppler shift versus time) at every point on a two-dimensional display. Instead, other techniques are used. Autocorrelation is the most common technique. With the use of autocorrelation, each echo is correlated with the corresponding echo from the previous pulse, thus determining the motion that has occurred during each pulse period. At least

three pulses per scan line are required to do this. A real-time value for mean flow speed is produced at each gate location along the scan line. As this is positive or negative with respect to flow direction, it is possible to present real-time, color-coded information on flow direction two-dimensionally on the display. Figure 2-12 shows flow in a vessel by using various color maps (color assignment schemes). On the left side of each display is a color map or color bar that shows the assignment of color to various mean Doppler shift frequencies. Figures 2-13A and B describe how this map includes various Doppler information (mean positive and negative Doppler shift values, wall filter region centered on the baseline, Nyquist limits, and variance). These aspects are all discussed below. The simplest color assignment (color map) is shown in Figure 2-12A. It assigns red to positive Doppler shifts and blue to negative shifts. Increasing the Doppler shift does not change the hue but increases its brightness. A slightly more complicated

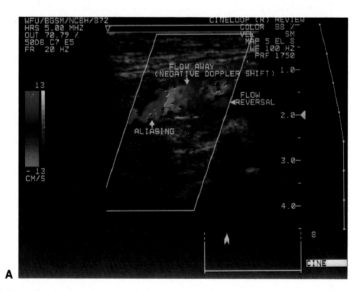

Fig. 2-12 Doppler shift and variance display. Flow is shown in a vessel indicating negative Doppler shifts (blue). The positive Doppler shifts (red) are due to flow reversal and to aliasing (see text). **(A)** Increasing positive and negative Doppler shifts progress from dark red to light red and from dark blue to light blue, respectively. (*Figure continues.*)

color map assigns red and blue as above but increases brightness and decreases saturation (i.e., approaches white) with increasing Doppler shift (Fig. 2-12B). The color map shown in Figure 2-12C changes hue as the Doppler shift increases (red progresses to yellow, i.e., green is added increasingly; blue progresses to cyan, i.e., green is added increasingly). In Figure 2-12D, red progresses to yellow and blue progresses to white. This is a combination of Figures 2-12B and C. The color assignments discussed above are based

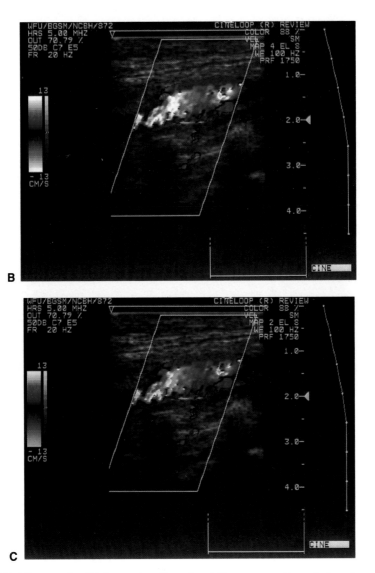

Fig. 2-12 (*Continued*). **(B)** Increasing Doppler shifts progress from dark red to white and from dark blue to white. **(C)** Increasing Doppler shifts progress from dark red to bright yellow and from dark blue to bright cyan. (*Figure continues.*)

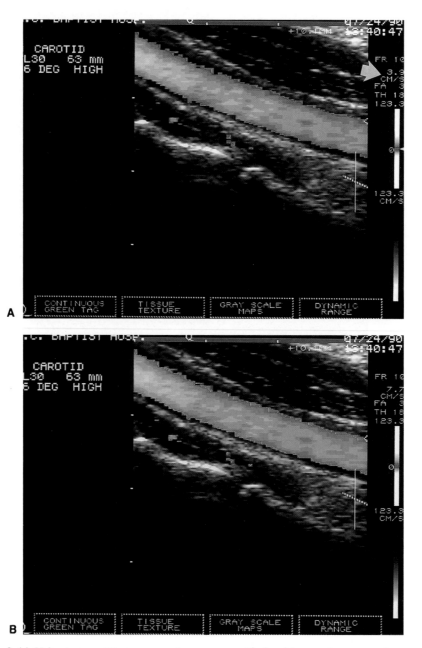

Fig. 2-14 Velocity tags. The green tag is set at a specific level (arrows) on an angle-corrected calibrated color bar. The green region on the display, therefore, indicates areas where that specific flow speed exists. (*Figure continues.*)

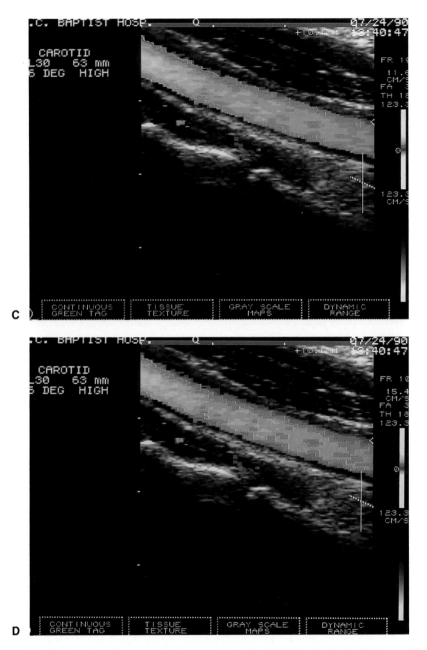

Fig. 2-14 (*Continued*). The green tag is set at **(A)** 3.9, **(B)** 7.7, **(C)** 11.6, **(D)** 15.4, **(E)** 19.3, **(F)** 23.1, **(G)** 27.0, **(H)** 30.8, and **(I)** 34.7 cm/s. As the set flow speed value increases, the indicated region (green) moves to the center, where the highest speed (30.8 cm/s) is found. A speed of 34.7 cm/s is not found anywhere in this scan (Fig. I). (*Figure continues.*)

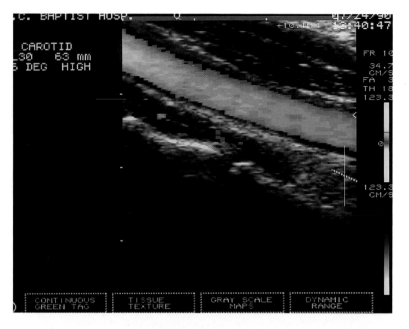

Fig. 2-14 (*Continued*).

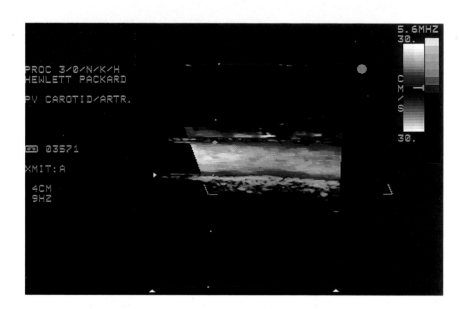

Fig. 2-15 Laminar flow. The color bar used in this scan progress from dark red and dark blue to bright white (decreasing saturation and increasing brightness). This presentation nicely shows laminar flow. The regions near the vessel wall are dark, with progressive brightening and decreasing saturation to white at the center left. This corresponds to the low flow speeds at the vessel wall and high flow speeds at the vessel center characteristic of laminar flow.

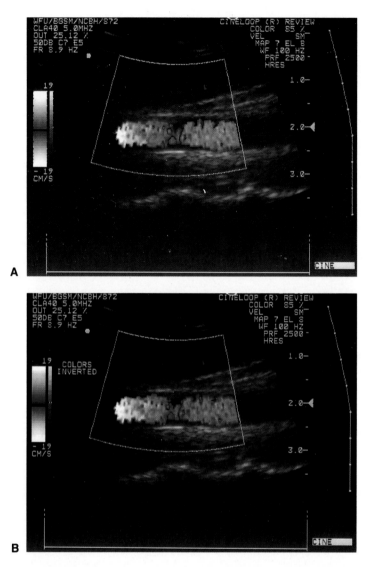

Fig. 2-16 Reversal of color assignment. Carotid artery flow imaged with a convex-array transducer. **(A)** Red indicates flow toward the transducer, and blue indicates flow away from the transducer; therefore, flow in this vessel is from right to left. **(B)** The blue and red assignments on the color map are reversed. Flow, of course, is still from right to left in the vessel, although the colors are reversed from those in Figure A. (Fig. B from Kremkau,[4] with permission.)

use of a green tag that identifies a specific value for Doppler shift or flow speed. For low values, regions near the vessel wall are identified. As the level increases, the appropriate regions are found progressively nearer the vessel center, where the highest value is found. This is an impressive presentation of normal laminar flow[2] in a vessel. A similar procedure can be used in which the green tag identifies all flow regions that exceed the set level. Figure 2-15 shows how a saturation map (red to white and blue to white) can nicely demonstrate laminar flow as well. The regions near the vessel wall are dark red (low flow speed) with progressive brightening to white at the center. Figure 2-16A shows an example of color inversion wherein red represents positive Doppler shift (approaching flow) and blue represents negative Doppler shift (receding flow). This has become the dominant color assignment in practice. In Figure 2-16B the color assignments are reversed.

A change in color from red to blue, or vice versa, can indicate a legitimate flow reversal or aliasing (Fig. 2-17). Aliasing is an artifact in pulsed-Doppler instruments[2] that also is exhibited in color-flow instruments because they too use the pulsed-Doppler technique. Aliasing results from a sampled frequency (Doppler shift) that is too high or a sampling frequency (pulse repetition frequency [PRF]) that is too low.[2,5] In a Doppler spectral display, aliasing results in Doppler presentation of incorrect direction. In a color-flow instrument this becomes presentation of the incorrect color (Fig. 2-18). As with spectral displays, aliasing can be decreased or eliminated by increasing the PRF (Fig. 2-19) or by shifting the baseline (Fig. 2-20). Aliasing occurs when the maximum Doppler shift frequency encountered exceeds one-half of the PRF. Thus, the maximum speed indicated at the extremes of the color maps represents a Doppler shift frequency equal to one-half the PRF (Figs. 2-5A and B, 2-13A, and 2-18A and B). This is called the *Nyquist limit* and can be presented in either hertz of Doppler shift (Fig. 2-5B) or centimeters per

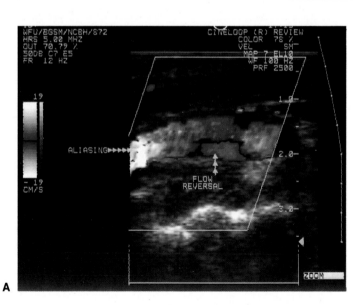

A

Fig. 2-17 Flow reversal versus aliasing. This scan shows true flow reversal in the carotid artery bulb, along with aliasing distal to it (flow is from right to left). The true flow reversal region is bounded by dark colors and black, representing the center of the color bar, the baseline, and the wall filter region. The aliasing boundary is represented in different ways depending on the color map. **(A)** The aliasing boundary is white because the map extremes are white; (*Figure continues.*)

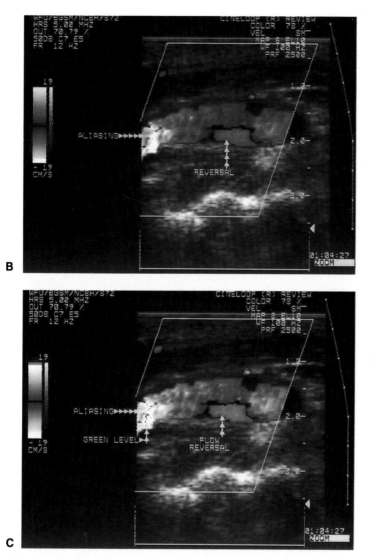

Fig. 2-17 (*Continued*). **(B)** the boundary is white and yellow, representing the map extremes; **(C)** the aliasing boundary is white, and the positive Nyquist limit is represented as green. On the scan, the green nicely shows the aliasing boundary.

second of flow speed (Fig. 2-5A), the latter being more common. Note that in Figure 2-5B the Nyquist limit is 625 Hz, (i.e., one-half of the displayed PRF, which is 1,250 Hz). When the Nyquist limit is exceeded, the presentation folds over to the other end of the color bar (Fig. 2-18). Continued increase of Doppler shift begins to show as a decrease in the wrong direction on the display. To differentiate between true flow reversal and aliasing, the boundary at the color change must be evaluated carefully. True flow reversal crosses the baseline through the wall filter (Fig. 2-13A) and has a dark boundary. Aliasing crosses from one map extreme to the other and has a bright boundary. Figure 2-17 shows the dark boundary around the true flow reversal in all three cases. With dif-

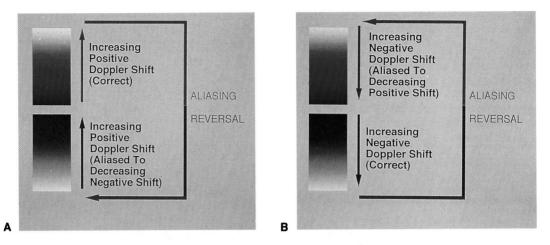

Fig. 2-18 Aliasing. The boxes on the left represent the positive and negative portions of the color map, with the wall filter separation in the center. **(A)** As the positive Doppler shift increases, the color representation moves up the upper half of the map until the Nyquist limit is reached. Increases in positive Doppler shift beyond this value produce aliasing and the color reversal to the bottom of the lower half of the map (the negative Nyquist limit). Increasing positive Doppler shifts beyond the Nyquist limit are aliased into decreasing negative shifts progressing toward the baseline. **(B)** As the Doppler shift (representing receding flow) increases, the color representation progresses down the lower half of the color bar to the Nyquist limit, where aliasing occurs and color reversal jumps to the top of the upper half of the color bar. Increasing negative Doppler shifts then are converted to decreasing positive shifts progressing toward the baseline.

ferent color maps, the alias boundary is presented differently. In Figure 2-17A the map extremes are white, so the alias boundary is white. In Figure 2-17B the blue goes to white and then aliases to yellow (Fig. 2-18B), continuing into red with increasing speed of receding flow. Here the increasing negative Doppler shift is aliased into a decreasing positive shift. In Figure 2-17C, blue goes to white and then aliases to white through a green value (maximum). The green then nicely delineates the aliasing boundary. No green or white is present around the flow reversal boundary.

Figure 2-21A shows a combined color-flow and gray-scale display; Figure 2-21B shows gray-scale display only, and Figure 2-21C shows color-flow display only. It is clear that the color-flow information is simply superimposed on the gray-scale image. Figure 2-22 shows the effect of the color gain control. As with gray-scale, increasing gain brightens the image. Time gain control (TGC) is applied to the color image in some instruments (Fig. 2-8D). The color map in Figure 2-17A can be modified to show when maximum positive Doppler shift is reached with green (Fig. 2-17C). This nicely identifies flow boundaries at which aliasing occurs.

Rather than showing each color frame individually, it is possible to average two or more consecutive frames. This process is called *smoothing* or *persistence* and it helps to fill in gaps in the presentation and present a

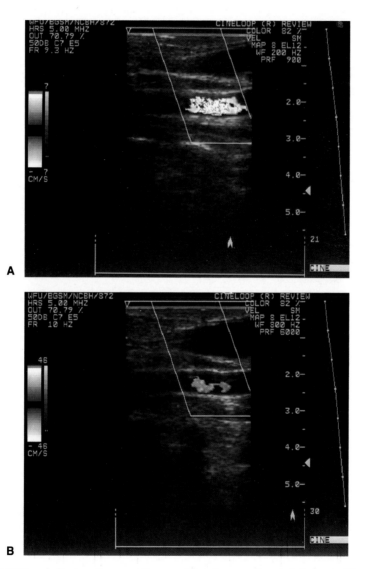

Fig. 2-19 PRF and aliasing. Lower pulse repetition frequencies result in lower Nyquist limits and a tendency toward aliasing. **(A)** The PRF is 900 Hz, and aliasing is occurring. **(B)** The PRF is 6,000 Hz, and the Nyquist limit has increased from 7 to 46 cm/s, which is sufficient to prevent aliasing at the velocities present in this vessel.

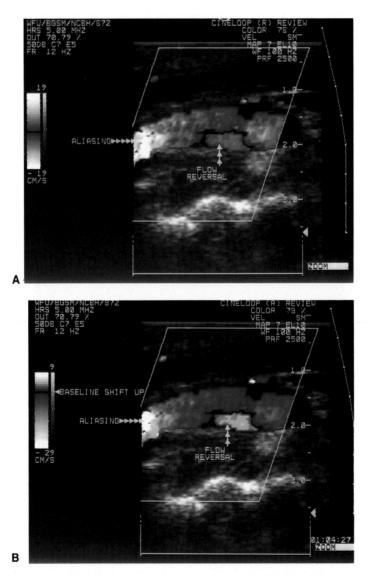

Fig. 2-20 Aliasing. **(A)** Aliasing is occurring in the left-hand side of the scan with a PRF of 2,500 Hz and a Nyquist limit of 19 cm/s. **(B)** The red portion of the aliasing region has been eliminated by shifting the baseline of the color bar up by 10 cm/s so that the positive Nyquist limit is 9 cm/s and the negative Nyquist limit is −29 cm/s. Note that the blue region has become darker and the flow reversal region has become brighter because of this baseline shift.

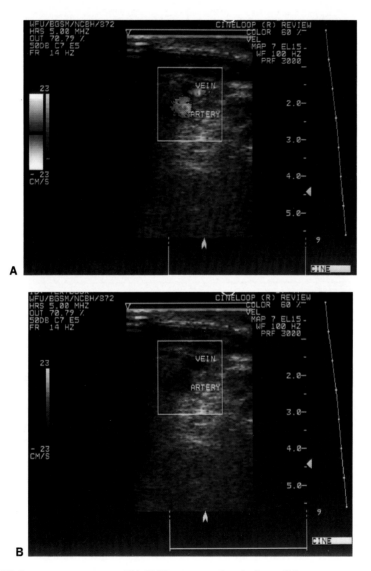

Fig. 2-21 Image components. **(A)** DCI cross-sectional view of the common carotid artery and jugular vein. If the cross-section were perpendicular to the flow, there would be no color in the vessels. **(B)** The color display is turned off. (*Figure continues.*)

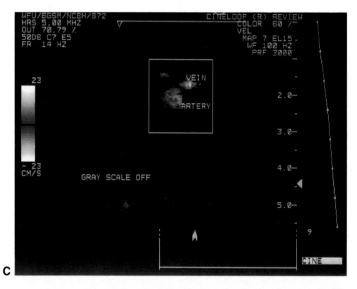

C

Fig. 2-21 (*Continued*). **(C)** The gray-scale display is turned off.

smoother but less detailed representation of flow (Fig. 2-23). A minimum of three pulses are required to generate a color scan line. The number of pulses per scan line is called the *ensemble length*. The greater the ensemble length, the better the detection of flow information (Fig. 2-23). However, because more pulses are required for each color scan line, the frame rate is reduced as the ensemble length is increased. On a display that has gray-scale information and color-flow information, both can be presented at each pixel location. More commonly, a decision is made to display gray or color but not both. With the latter approach, sometimes control is provided over the priority given to color or gray (Fig. 2-24).

Wall motion in the heart or the pulsing arteries and tissue motion can produce low-frequency, high-amplitude Doppler shifts that can clutter the image with unwanted motion information (Figs. 2-25A and B). Wall filters are provided that eliminate Doppler shift frequencies below their set threshold but permit the passage of higher frequencies. These are adjustable, allowing the elimination of wall motion artifacts (Fig. 2-25C). To reduce aliasing, PRF must be increased. To detect slow flows, PRF must be decreased. The frame rate (number of color images produced per second) depends on the PRF, imaging depth, color window width, and ensemble number:

$$FR = \frac{PRF}{LPF \times EL}$$

where FR is the frame rate, LPF is the number of scan lines in the color window, and EL is the ensemble length (number of pulses per color scan line). Increasing the color window width increases the number of scan lines contained in the window. The imaging depth limits the PRF because all echoes from a pulse must be received before the next pulse can be emitted.[1] Thus, greater imaging depths reduce PRF and FR. Figure 2-26 illustrates the effect of increasing color window width

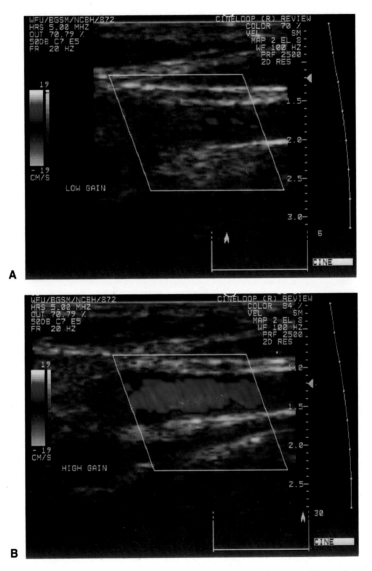

Fig. 2-22 Color gain. Increasing color gain increases the brightness of the color presentation.
(A) Low color gain (70%) and **(B)** high color gain (84%) are shown.

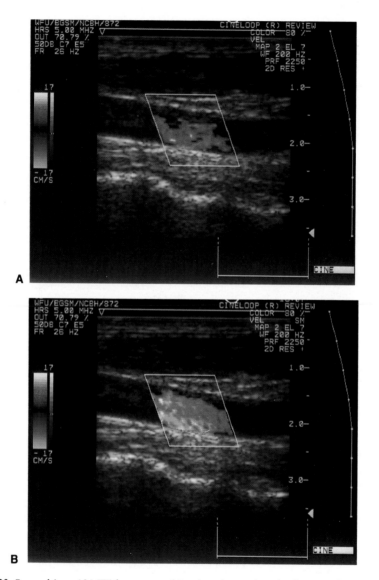

Fig. 2-23 Smoothing. **(A)** With no smoothing (persistence), only the Doppler-shifted echoes received from the pulses generating an individual frame are shown. **(B)** With smoothing, consecutive frames are averaged, filling gaps in the presentation and presenting a smoother but less detailed representation of flow. (*Figure continues.*)

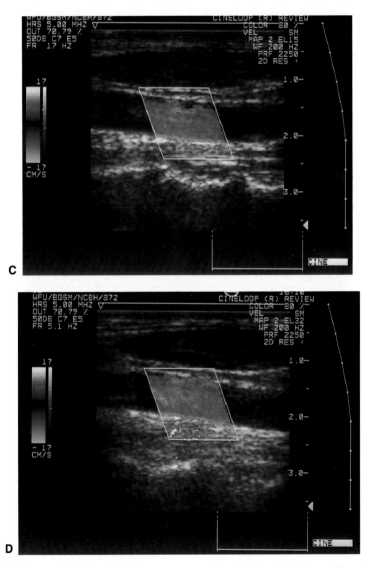

Fig. 2-23 (*Continued*). **(C & D)** More accurate and complete detection of flow information is obtained with increasing ensemble lengths. The ensemble lengths shown are Fig. B, 7; Fig. C, 15; and Fig. D, 32. Note the decrease in frame rate from 26 to 17 to 5.1 frames per second.

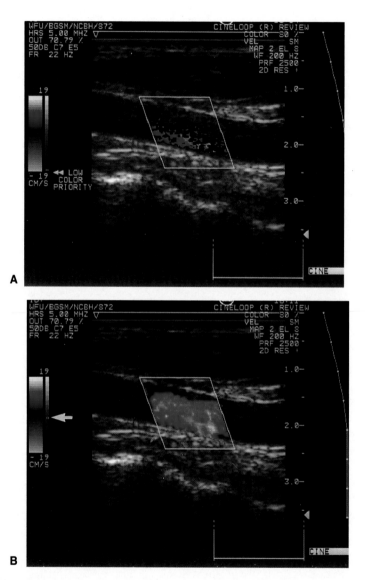

Fig. 2-24 Color write priority. **(A)** With the color priority set low (at the bottom of the gray bar), weak, non-Doppler-shifted reverberation and off-axis echoes within the vessel take precedence over the Doppler-shifted echoes, and little color is displayed. **(B)** With a higher priority, halfway up the gray bar (arrow), the Doppler-shifted echoes (color) take precedence over the weaker gray-scale echoes.

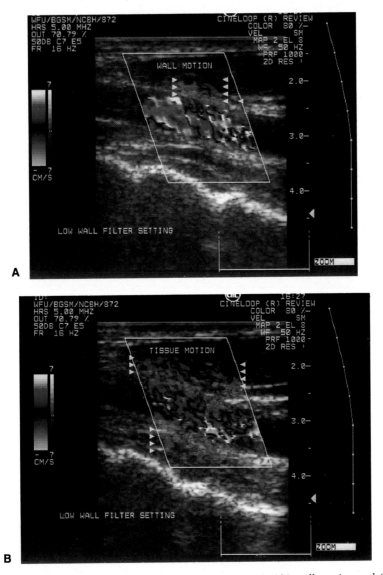

Fig. 2-25 Wall filters. With a low wall filter setting (50 Hz), **(A)** wall motion and **(B)** tissue motion appear in color on the image. (*Figure continues.*)

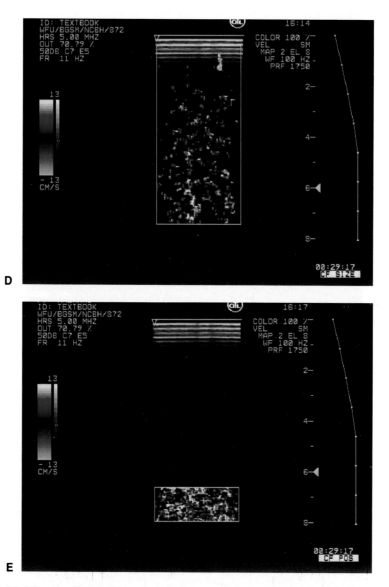

Fig. 2-26 (*Continued*). **(D)** The color window extends to a depth of nearly 8 cm. **(E)** Shortening the color window to cover a smaller region does not decrease the frame rate (11 Hz) in Figs. D and E. This is because the instrument must wait just as long for the deep echoes to arrive in both cases regardless of whether the earlier echoes are imaged.

on frame rate. Figure 2-23 illustrates the effect of ensemble length on frame rate.

Some instruments continually store the last several (e.g., 32) frames imaged and permit the user to show any one of them individually after the image has been frozen. Figures 2-26A to C show frames 12, 30, and 30, respectively, of the last 32 acquired in each case (see the lower right corner of each image).

Other details of Doppler instruments can be found elsewhere.[2,4,6–9]

ARTIFACTS

In diagnostic ultrasonography, perhaps more than in any other imaging method, artifacts are of great clinical importance. Each form of ultrasonography is associated with its own unique artifacts. These have been described most extensively with respect to B-mode and Doppler systems. Many artifacts are induced by errors in scanning technique (such as failure to image at an acceptable angle) or instrument setup (improper gain producing artificial echoes within a cyst, causing it to be regarded as solid, or vice versa) and are therefore preventable. The importance of artifacts in influencing interpretation is that they may suggest the presence of structures that are not actually present, causing misdiagnosis, or they may cause important findings to be obscured. In addition, they may alter the size, shape, or brightness of structures.[1,10,11] Although generally an impediment to accurate interpretation of the image, some artifacts may aid in diagnosis. Since the understanding of artifacts is so important in the correct interpretation of ultrasound examinations and since many artifacts can be prevented by careful imaging techniques, discussion of artifacts related to DCI is appropriate. In general, artifacts that alter ultrasound interpretation may be classified as follows:

1. Artifacts that suggest the presence of structures not actually present
2. Artifacts that remove real echoes from the display or obscure information
3. Artifacts that distort the size, shape, or brightness of a structure (displacement of echoes on the display from their proper location)
4. Artifacts that impair the accurate estimation of hemodynamic parameters including flow direction, velocity, and turbulence

Artifacts observed in DCI are color presentations of artifacts that traditionally have been seen in gray-scale imaging and Doppler spectral displays.[11] Although many of the problems and artifacts associated with B-mode imaging, such as shadowing, are encountered with duplex Doppler and DCI, the detection and display of frequency information related to moving targets add a group of special artifacts not encountered when other forms of ultrasonography are used. An understanding of these artifacts and their influence on the interpretation of flow measurements obtained in clinical practice is important.

The most important artifacts encountered when using DCI include effects due to Doppler angle, aliasing, shadowing, clutter, grating lobes, mirror, and range ambiguity. Figures 2-17, 2-19, 2-20, and 2-27 give examples of color aliasing and its elimination with increasing PRF or with baseline shifts. Figure 2-28 illustrates the lack of color information when the Doppler angle is zero. Figure 2-16 shows color reversal due to a changing Doppler angle with sector scan lines from a convex array. One would not expect such a color reversal in a straight vessel with a linear array. However, in Figure 2-29 the unexpected appears. Here the flow reversal is a normal physiologic event occurring briefly in diastole. Forward and reverse flows are both shown in the image because the right

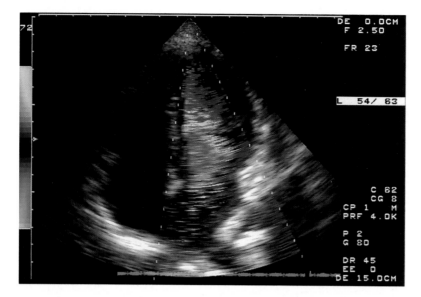

Fig. 2-27 Aliasing and depth. In this color-flow image of the heart, all flow is toward the transducer even though a color reversal is seen. The flow should all appear red, but in the lower portion it has aliased to blue because the Nyquist limit has been exceeded.

and left sides of the image are produced at different times. In this case 78 ms has elapsed during generation of the image, permitting imaging of late systole and early diastolic flow reversal simultaneously. Figure 2-30A illustrates shadowing in a color scan. Note that the shadowing for the gray scale follows the scan lines, whereas for the color window the shadowing is at an angle following the color scan lines. Figure 2-30B illustrates grating lobes[1,11] in a phased linear array. A grating lobe is an additional beam that propagates in a different direction than the primary beam from an array transducer. The instrument assumes that all echoes are from the primary beam and places them along the scan line that corresponds to the assumed path of the primary beam. This placement is incorrect for the grating lobe echoes. Mirror image similar to that observed in gray-scale imaging[1,2] can also be observed during color-flow imaging (Fig. 2-31).[12,13] Range ambiguity encountered in gray-scale imaging[1] and in pulsed Doppler[14] can also occur in color-flow imaging. Color may appear artifactually in an-

echoic regions without flow due to noise or tissue motion.[13,15] Figure 2-30C illustrates clutter resulting from relative motion between a transducer and a calculus in the bladder of a cat. Perivascular tissue vibration caused by turbulent intravascular blood flow can produce artifactual extravascular color presentation.[16]

SAFETY

Experience with diagnostic ultrasound to date has shown no hazards to patients or users. The Statement on Ultrasound Bioeffects of the American Institute of Ultrasound in Medicine (AIUM) (see p. 58) notes that although the possibility that biologic effects might be identified in the future, "the benefits to patients of the prudent use of diagnostic ultrasound outweigh the risks, if any, that may be present."[17] Although reassuring, this statement raises several issues that must be considered by users of diagnostic ultrasound as knowledge of the bioeffects of ul-

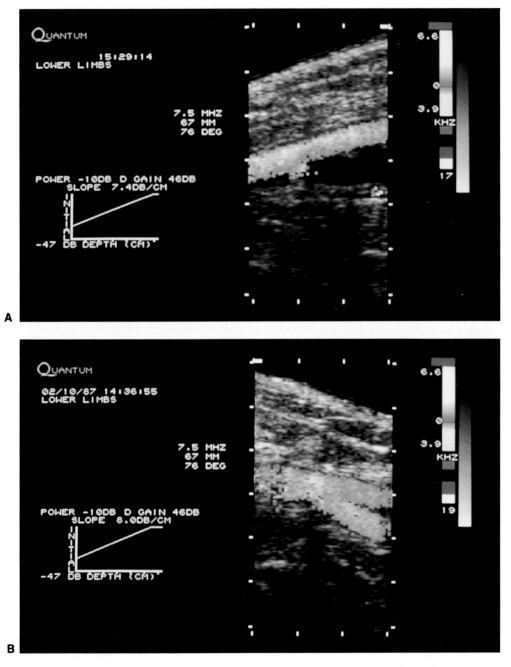

Fig. 2-28 Doppler angle flow artifact. **(A)** The common and superficial femoral arteries are seen, but the profunda femoral artery appears to have no flow (no color within it). **(B)** With the use of a suitable Doppler angle, flow is shown in all vessels including the profunda femoral artery. The 90-degree Doppler angle in Fig. A causes no Doppler shift and lack of color. (From Kremkau,[2] with permission.)

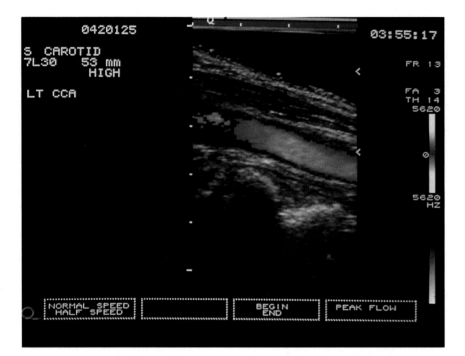

Fig. 2-29 Physiologic change in flow direction. This image of the common carotid artery shows flow from left to right. On the right and left sides of the image the flow is reversed. The relationship of the scan lines and the vessel is constant, eliminating a change of Doppler angle as an explanation of the color change. Here the image has captured a physiologic reversal of flow in diastole. Since the generation of the entire image frame requires from 50 to 100 ms depending on the frame rate, a single image may display dynamic changes in flow that occur during that interval.

trasound increases and new applications of ultrasound such as DCI are introduced into routine clinical practice. All physicians accept the obligation to protect their patients from unnecessary harm and therefore should attempt to provide maximum benefit with minimal risk. To meet these obligations for patient safety, the user should implement the common-sense principle of "as low as reasonably achievable" (ALARA).[18,19] Under the principle of ALARA, users are encouraged to keep exposure to levels that are as low as reasonably achievable in keeping with diagnostic objectives.

Two potential mechanisms for producing bi-ologic effects by ultrasound are currently understood. These include thermal mechanisms, which result from tissue heating owing to the absorption of ultrasound as it passes through tissue, and nonthermal (mechanical) effects such as cavitation and radiation force. Cavitation refers to the formation and collapse of microbubbles around cavitation nuclei. The extent to which these nuclei exist in normal tissue is unclear. Currently thermal mechanisms are better understood than nonthermal mechanisms with respect to their relationship to bioeffects. Thermal and mechanical mechanisms are each capable of producing biologic effects at high levels.

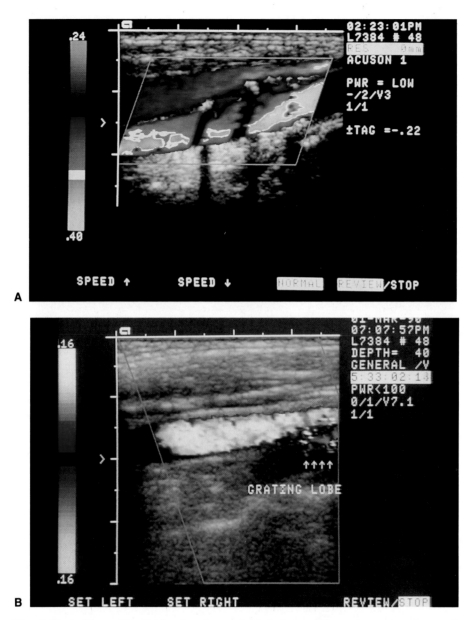

Fig. 2-30 Artifacts. **(A)** Shadowing from calcified plaque follows the gray-scale scan lines straight down while following the angled color scan lines parallel to the sides of the parallelogram. **(B)** Grating-lobe artifact appears as an incorrect color (blue), slightly outside the vessel on this scan. The primary beam pulses parallel the scan lines that are directed 20 degrees to the right. However, the grating lobe travels to the left, encountering receding flow, and presents it along the primary beam scan lines as negative Doppler shift (blue). (*Figure continues.*)

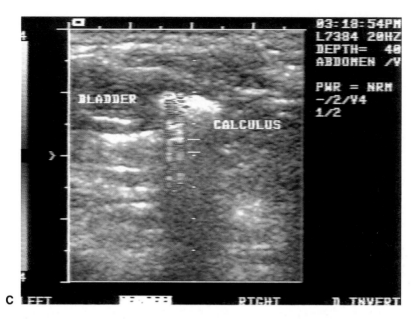

Fig. 2-30 (*Continued*). (**C**) Color echoes are present in the shadow region below the calculus in the bladder of a cat. Relative motion between the transducer and the calculus may have produced these echoes. The mechanism of this artifact is not clear.

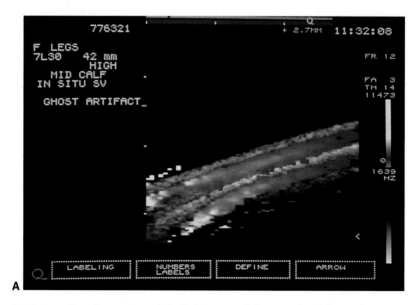

Fig. 2-31 Reverberation artifact. (**A**) This image of the superficial femoral artery is accompanied by a ghost image deep to the vessel. (*Figure continues.*)

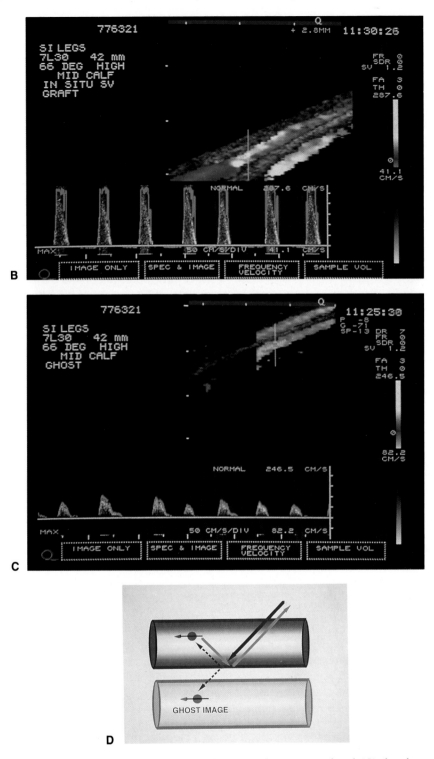

Fig. 2-31 (*Continued*). Spectral sampling from (**B**) the true vessel and (**C**) the ghost vessel reveals similar signals. (**D**) The ghost image results when echoes from moving red cells within the artery are delayed in their return (dotted line) by a multiple-path reflection from the vessel wall. The delay in the return of these echoes is assumed by the machine to indicate a greater distance of the target from the transducer, so the false image is displayed deep to the true vessel.

Ultrasound devices may operate in several modes, including real-time imaging, DCI, spectral Doppler, and M-mode. Pulsed ultrasound is used for real-time imaging, spectral Doppler, and color Doppler applications. The nature of the ultrasound pulses and the resulting acoustic exposure differ significantly among these operating modes, resulting in important bioeffects considerations. Imaging is produced in a scanned mode of operation (Fig. 2-1A). In scanned modes, pulses of ultrasound from the transducer are directed down lines of sight that are moved or steered in sequence to generate the image. This means that the number of ultrasound pulses arriving at a given point in the patient over a given time interval is relatively small and that relatively little energy is deposited at any given location. By contrast, Doppler is an unscanned mode of operation in which multiple ultrasound pulses are sent in repetition along a line to collect the Doppler data (Fig. 2-1B). In this mode the beam is stationary, resulting in considerably greater potential for heating than in imaging modes. For imaging, the frequency at which the pulses are emitted (the PRF) is usually a few kilohertz, with very short pulses. With both duplex and color Doppler, longer pulse durations are used than with imaging. In addition, to avoid aliasing and other artifacts when using Doppler, it is often necessary to user higher PRFs than those used in imaging applications.

As a class, Doppler instruments have the highest outputs observed in diagnostic ultrasound.[2,20,21] However, color Doppler instruments have lower outputs than pulsed duplex Doppler instruments. Longer pulse duration and higher PRF result in higher duty factors for Doppler modes of operation and increase the amount of energy introduced in scanning. Color Doppler, although a scanned mode, produces exposure conditions between those of real-time imaging and Doppler because color Doppler devices tend to send more pulses down each scan line and may use longer pulse durations than imaging devices. Clearly, every user should be aware that when switching from an imaging to a Doppler mode, the exposure conditions and potential for bioeffects change.

With current devices operating in imaging modes, bioeffects concerns are minimal because intensities sufficient to produce measurable heating are seldom used. This statement is probably true for most DCI operating modes as well. With pulsed spectral Doppler, however, the potential for thermal effects is greater.

In obstetric applications the need for prudent use is particularly important. Users should attempt to prevent unnecessary exposure and refrain from performing examinations under high-exposure conditions unless they are truly clinically warranted. Examiner skill and experience are important to permit efficient collection of diagnostic information with minimal exposure.

Although the use of diagnostic ultrasound carries no known risk, prudent practice dictates that color Doppler ultrasound be used for medical indications with the minimum exposure time and instrument output required to obtain the needed diagnostic information.[1,17,21] Output information is beginning to be provided in real-time (Fig. 2-32). This information assists the operator in the implementation of ALARA and will become generally available in the near future. Standards are being developed for display of this information as a joint effort between several professional societies involved in ultrasound, instrument manufacturers, and the federal government.

SUMMARY

DCI acquires Doppler-shifted echoes from a cross-section of tissue scanned by an ultrasound beam. These echoes are then presented in color and superimposed on the gray-scale anatomic image of non-Doppler-shifted echoes received during the scan. The flow echoes are assigned colors according to the color map chosen. Usually red, yellow, or white indicates positive Doppler shifts (approaching flow) and blue, cyan, or white indicates negative shifts (receding flow). Green is added to indicate variance (disturbed or turbulent flow). Several pulses (the number is called the ensemble length) are needed to generate a color scan line. Linear, convex, phased, and annular arrays are used to acquire the gray-scale and color-flow information. Doppler color-flow instruments are pulsed-Doppler instruments and are subject to the same limitations, such as Doppler angle dependence and aliasing, as other Doppler instruments. Color controls include gain, TGC, map selection, variance on/off, persistence, ensemble length, color/gray

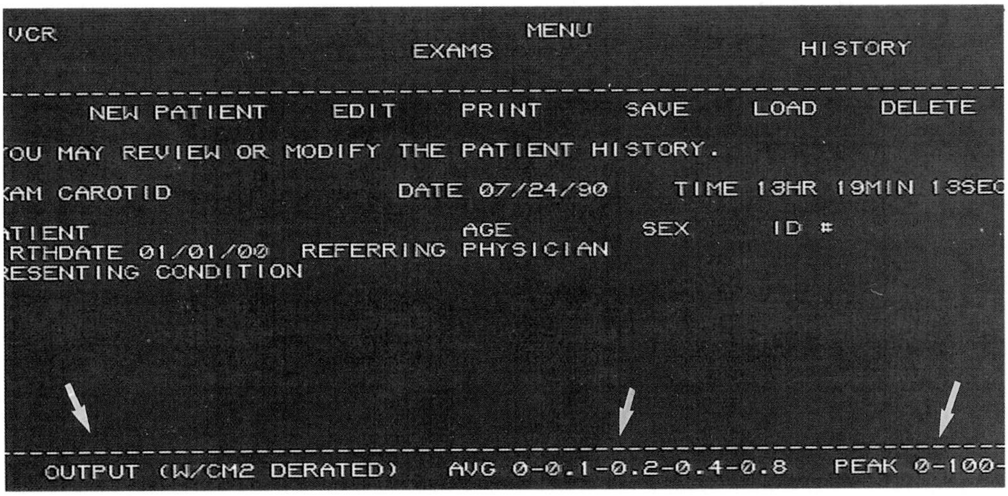

Fig. 2-32 Acoustic output display. Some instrument displays now include output power information. On this instrument, average and peak output intensities based on assumed tissue attenuation are presented (arrows).

priority, Nyquist limit (PRF), baseline shift, wall filter, and color window angle, location, and size. Doppler color-flow instruments generally have output intensities intermediate between those of gray-scale imaging and pulsed-Doppler duplex instruments. Although there is no known risk with the use of color-flow instruments, prudent practice dictates that they be used for medical indications and with the minimum exposure time and instrument output required to obtain the needed diagnostic information.

ACKNOWLEDGMENTS

We gratefully acknowledge the assistance of John Allison, Cynthia Burnham, Diane Branscome, Robert Kaylor, Marie King, Anne Mansfield, Chris Merritt, Paul Ramsey, Pam Rowland, Dennis Shields, Jackie Sledge, Kathy Spaulding, and Paul Tesh. We also thank the following companies: Acuson, Advanced Technology Laboratories, Diasonics, Hewlett-Packard, and Quantum Medical Systems for assistance in generating scans for figures. The efforts of Kim Eldridge in manuscript preparation are also acknowledged with appreciation.

REFERENCES

1. Kremkau FW: Diagnostic Ultrasound: Principles, Instruments, and Exercises. 3rd Ed. WB Saunders, Philadelphia, 1989
2. Kremkau FW: Doppler Ultrasound: Principles and Instruments. WB Saunders, Philadelphia, 1990
3. Kremkau FW: Modern transducer terminology. J Diagn Med Sonogr 6:293, 1990
4. Kremkau FW: Principles of color flow imaging. J Vasc Technol 15:104, 265, 325, 1991
5. Kremkau FW: Doppler artifacts. J Vasc Technol 14:41, 123, 239, 1991
6. Kremkau FW: Doppler principles. Semin Roentgenol 27:1, 1992
7. Evans DH, McDicken WN, Skidmore R, Woodcock JP: Doppler Ultrasound: Physics, Instrumentation, and Clinical Applications. John Wiley & Sons, New York, 1989
8. Kremkau FW: Principles and pitfalls of real-time color-flow imaging. In Bernstein EF (ed): Vascular Diagnosis. Mosby-Year Book, St. Louis, (in press)
9. Kasai C, Namekawa K, Koyano A, Omoto R: Real-time two-dimensional blood flow imaging using an autocorrelation technique. IEEE Trans Sonics Ultrasonics SU-32:458, 1985
10. Powis RL, Powis WJ (eds): Artifacts we should know. p. 379. In A Thinker's Guide to Ultrasonic Imaging. Urban and Schwartzenberg, Baltimore, 1984
11. Kremkau FW, Taylor KJW: Artifacts in ultrasound imaging. J Ultrasound Med 5:227, 1986
12. Reading CC, Charboneau JW, Allison JW, Cooperberg PL: Color and spectral Doppler mirror-image artifact of the subclavian artery. Radiology 174:41, 1990
13. Middleton WD, Melson GL: The carotid ghost. A color Doppler ultrasound duplication artifact. J Ultrasound Med 9:487, 1990
14. Gill RW, Kossoff G, Griffiths KA: New class of pulsed Doppler US ambiguity at short ranges. Radiology 173:272, 1989
15. Mitchell DG, Burns P, Needleman L: Color Doppler artifacts in anechoic regions. J Ultrasound Med 9:255, 1990
16. Middleton WD, Erickson S, Melson GL: Perivascular color artifact: pathologic significance and appearance on color Doppler US images. Radiology 171:647, 1989
17. American Institute of Ultrasound in Medicine: Bioeffects considerations for the safety of diagnostic ultrasound. J Ultrasound Med 7(suppl):S4, 1988
18. National Council on Radiation Protection and Measurements: NCRP Report No. 107. Implementation of the Principle of As Low as Reasonably Achievable (ALARA) for Medical and Dental Personnel. National Council on Radiation Protection and Measurements, Bethesda, MD, 1990
19. Merritt CRB: Safety Issues in Diagnostic Ultrasound. Categorical Course in Ultrasound. Radiological Society of North America, Oak Brook, IL, 1991
20. Taylor KJW, Kremkau FW: Diminishing exposure to Doppler ultrasound. The sonographer's role. J Diagn Med Sonogr 4:5, 1988
21. Kremkau FW: Biological effects and safety. p. 19. In Rumack CM, Wilson SR, Charboneau JW (eds): Diagnostic Ultrasound. Mosby-Year Book, St. Louis, 1991

3

Carotid and Vertebral Arteries

Edward I. Bluth
Christopher R. B. Merritt

Stroke is a significant public health problem. It is currently the third leading cause of mortality in the United States and is responsible for more than 200,000 deaths per year. In addition, with modern medical therapies, three times this number of stroke victims survive with some residual impairment. The value of a safe, noninvasive, and low-cost screening test for conditions that predispose to stroke is therefore great. Duplex Doppler ultrasonography combining high-resolution imaging and Doppler spectrum analysis is currently the test that best meets these goals. Over the past decade, numerous studies[1-3] have shown duplex sonography to be an effective and accurate means of assessing and detecting arteriosclerotic disease at the carotid bifurcation. Although duplex Doppler is recognized as highly reliable in the detection of significant stenosis of the extracranial carotid circulation, in some patients duplex examinations are difficult and, occasionally, misleading results are obtained. Some of the problems encountered with duplex Doppler have been successfully dealt with by the introduction of Doppler color imaging (DCI),

an important and highly useful adjunct to duplex Doppler in the evaluation of the carotid vessels. Several recent reports[4-8] have confirmed the value of DCI in assessment of the carotid and vertebral arteries. As in other applications, DCI does not replace spectral analysis but complements it.

Prior to the introduction of duplex and DCI, evaluation for the risk of stroke centered on identifying flow-limited stenosis by oculoplethysmography, periorbital bidirectional Doppler, and conventional or digital arteriography. Identification of flow-limiting stenosis is important because two-thirds of strokes result from arteriosclerotic stenosis, particularly in the region of the carotid bifurcation. With high-grade stenosis or occlusion, hemodynamic factors and low perfusion pressure probably contribute to symptoms. In addition, the presence of high-grade internal carotid stenosis, even in the absence of symptoms, is considered by many to be associated with increased risk for transient ischemic attack (TIA), stroke, and carotid occlusion.

Embolic disease is another significant cause of stroke; it sometimes is associated with arteriosclerotic disease of the carotid bifurcation. In fact, it is estimated that 50 to 60 percent of patients with TIAs have less than 50 percent stenosis on arteriography. It is known that certain carotid plaques develop hemorrhage and ulceration. Resulting endothelial damage may cause plaque debris and thrombus to be discharged into the vessel and travel distally, leading to embolic stroke. With high-resolution imaging, intraplaque hemorrhage can be identified, permitting plaque characterization and aiding in determining the relative risk for embolic complications.

PRINCIPLES AND INSTRUMENTATION

To use DCI successfully in cerebrovascular evaluation, the examiner must have an appreciation of carotid vascular anatomy and a thorough knowledge of examination techniques. A standardized and systematic method for evaluating the carotid and vertebral vessels should be employed. The examiner must be familiar with a variety of abnormal findings and their classification. In addition, an understanding of the Doppler principles and instrumentation summarized in Chapter 2 is essential to obtain maximum benefit from the information provided by DCI in the peripheral arterial system. Throughout the study, the examiner must be aware of the compromises required to obtain the best images of the vessel wall and plaque and the most accurate Doppler measurements. The best gray-scale images of vessel walls and plaque are obtained when the ultrasound beam is perpendicular to the vessel wall, whereas Doppler sampling requires an angle of 45 to 60 degrees between the sound beam and the direction of flow being sampled. When the Doppler angle is greater than 70 degrees, progressively smaller frequency shifts are observed and accurate estimation

of velocity is prevented. When the Doppler beam is perpendicular to the direction of blood flow, no Doppler shift is detected, leading to the impression that flow is absent.

With DCI, variations in the Doppler frequency shift resulting from changes in the Doppler angle produce changes in color saturation that may suggest changes in flow velocity if the angle of insonation to the presumed direction of flow is not closely observed and taken into account. This is particularly likely to be a problem when the vessels under examination are tortuous or make abrupt changes in direction relative to the transducer. Fortunately, global sampling of Doppler data with DCI makes it easier to observe the true course of tortuous vessels than with gray-scale alone. When a tortuous vessel makes a sharp turn, abruptly decreasing the Doppler angle, the resultant false velocity shift can be more easily identified than with duplex instruments because with DCI the direction of flow at each point in the vessel can be estimated (Fig. 3-1). Thus with DCI, more precise estimation of the Doppler angle is possible, permitting more accurate velocity estimation.[9,10]

The combination of high scanning frequencies and the relatively high flow velocities encountered in the carotid arteries, especially in the presence of significant stenosis, may result in aliasing of the Doppler signal (Fig. 3-2). As discussed in Chapter 2, it is important to recognize the appearance of aliasing with DCI; when present, this appearance is a useful indicator of high Doppler frequency shifts that may indicate stenosis.

ANATOMY

In most patients, the right common carotid artery arises from the right innominate artery. The left common carotid artery arises most commonly directly from the aortic arch. Anomalies of the common carotid

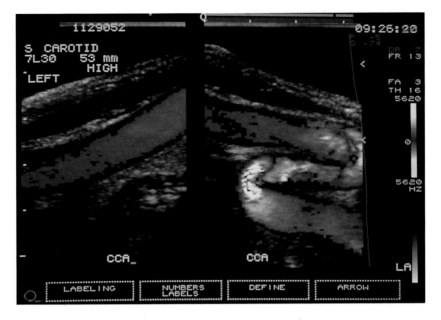

Fig. 3-1 Tortuous CCA. Flow is from right to left in this image of the CCA. Although there is no stenosis, note the change in color saturation and color reversal in the ascending loop of the vessel. This indicates a large Doppler frequency shift resulting from a Doppler angle near 0 degrees. By noticing that the vessel walls are completely filled with color, the examiner can be assured that the vessel is simply tortuous and not significantly stenosed.

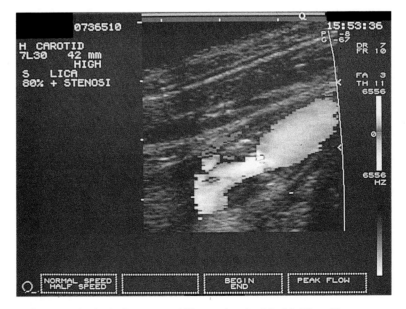

Fig. 3-2 Aliasing. The high-frequency shift associated with this 70 to 80 percent stenosis of the ICA exceeds the Nyquist limit, and the highest frequencies in the stenotic jet are displayed in light blue, rather than red, even though flow is not reversed. With DCI, aliasing appears as a continuation of the color scale from the shades used to display the highest positive frequency shifts to those used to display the greatest negative shifts. Chapter 2 provides a detailed explanation of the DCI display of aliasing.

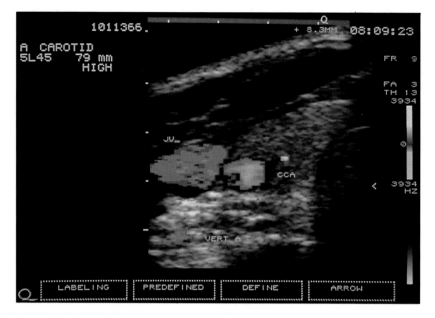

Fig. 3-3 Normal CCA. Transverse scan at the level of the mid-thyroid demonstrating the CCA bulb (red) medial to the larger jugular vein (blue). The vertebral artery (red) is posterior to the jugular vein. A small area of normal flow reversal is seen along the lateral wall of the CCA.

origins are not uncommon. In 10 to 20 percent of patients, the right innominate artery and the left common carotid artery may have a common origin. Other less common anomalies include the right common carotid artery originating directly from the aortic arch and the left common carotid artery originating directly from the left subclavian artery. In general, these anomalous origins have little effect on the duplex carotid examination. However, with arterial occlusion, unusual collateral flow may develop because of these anomalous origins.

In most patients, the carotid artery is medial to the jugular vein (Fig. 3-3). The common carotid artery (CCA) can generally be easily distinguished from the jugular vein by noting its pulsatility, flow direction, smaller size, and lack of compressibility as compared with the jugular vein. The carotid bifurcation is typically located at the level of the fourth cervical vertebra. However, it may be located as low as T2 or as high as C1. In general, low bifurcations are not a problem for sonographic evaluation. On the other hand, high bifurcations may be difficult to image as well because of the angle of the mandible. In such situations, positioning the transducer posteriorly is the most effective means of imaging the high bifurcation. In the vast majority of patients, the proximal internal carotid artery (ICA) is located posterior and lateral to the external carotid artery (ECA) (Fig. 3-4). This is a very useful feature in distinguishing these two vessels. On occasion, this relationship between the internal and external carotid artery is reversed; in such cases, other criteria may be used to distinguish the two vessels. One morphologic difference between the two vessels that can be detected more easily by DCI is the presence of branches arising from the external carotid artery (Fig. 3-5).

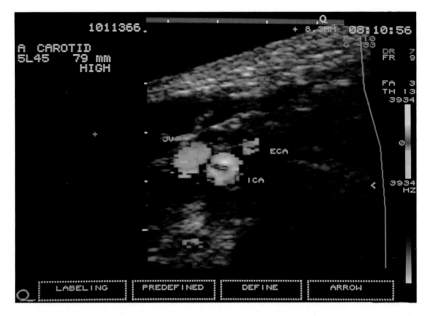

Fig. 3-4 ICA and ECA. Transverse scan beyond the carotid bifurcation shows the ICA posterior and lateral to the smaller ECA. The jugular vein (blue) is anterior, and the vertebral artery (red) is posterior.

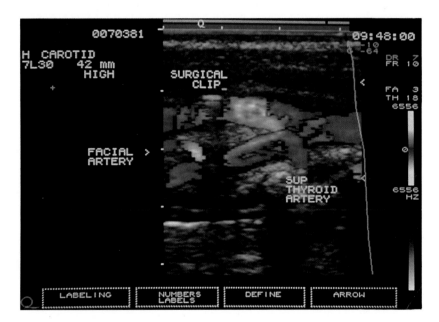

Fig. 3-5 External carotid branches. Sagittal scan shows the superior thyroid artery arising from near the origin of the external carotid artery and the facial artery further distally. Visible branches of the ECA include the superior thyroid, lingual, and facial arteries. The presence of such branches is easily shown by DCI and aids in differentiation of the ECA from the ICA, which has no branches at this level.

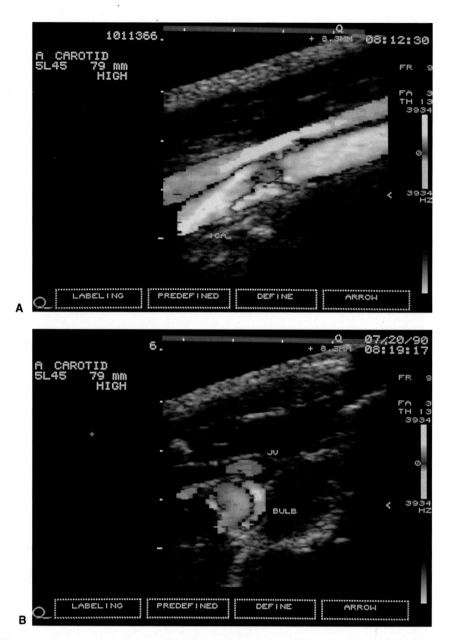

Fig. 3-6 Flow reversal. **(A)** Longitudinal and **(B)** transverse images of the carotid bifurcation reveal a localized area of reversed flow (blue) along the wall of the carotid bulb opposite the origin of the ECA. This is a normal finding. The carotid vessels are posterior to the jugular vein (blue).

The carotid artery widens just proximal to its bifurcation at the bulb. Depending on the level of the bifurcation, usually several centimeters of the proximal internal and external carotid arteries can be visualized. When DCI is used, a normal flow reversal (Fig. 3-6) is noted at the bulb. This is located peripherally, usually at the side opposite to the origin of the external carotid artery (ECA).

INDICATIONS FOR CAROTID ULTRASOUND

Since the primary purpose of noninvasive screening is to identify potentially treatable lesions in patients at increased risk for stroke, it is reasonable to consider as potential candidates for screening with ultrasound all patients with risk factors for stroke. Common indications for carotid ultrasonography are shown in Table 3-1.

Table 3-1 Common Indications for Carotid Ultrasonography

Patients with known arteriosclerotic cardiovascular disease, including
  Patients with peripheral vascular occlusive disease
  Patients with coronary artery disease
  Coronary bypass candidates

Patients with cardiac impairment, including
  Left ventricular hypertrophy
  Poor cardiac function

History of TIAs or symptoms of cerebrovascular insufficiency

History of equivocal or questionable symptoms of cerebrovascular insufficiency

Hypertension

Diabetes

Presence of other risk factors associated with atherosclerotic disease, including family history

Asymptomatic bruit

Endarterectomy—intraoperative and postoperative assessment

EXAMINATION TECHNIQUE

The examination is performed with the patient supine. The examiner can evaluate the patient by sitting either at the level of the patient's shoulders facing the patient, or above the patient and reaching over the patient's head to the neck. In any case, it is very important that both examiner and patient be comfortable since the examination usually takes 20 to 30 minutes (Fig. 3-7). For best access to the structures of interest, the patient's neck must be hyperextended. Depending on the patient, the carotid vessels can be found by scanning the neck with the chin straight or turned away from the side of the vessel being examined. On occasion, the vessels are best approached by scanning from posterior rather than anterior to the sternocleidomastoid muscles. At times both approaches are necessary to evaluate the vessels completely (Fig. 3-8).

To gain maximal benefit from the combined tissue and flow imaging capabilities of DCI, it is valuable to conduct the carotid examination in two parts. The examination is begun by using gray-scale imaging only, with careful examination of the vessel wall for evidence of intimal thickening and plaque. The highest possible imaging frequency should be used. When plaque is encountered, longitudinal and transverse imaging should be performed in an effort to characterize the plaque as homogeneous or heterogeneous. Flow imaging should then be added, with thorough inspection of the vessel for areas of flow disturbance, turbulence, or velocity changes indicating stenosis. Finally, spectral Doppler recordings are made at sites within the CCA, ICA, and ECA, as well as at sites of disturbed flow.

It is easiest to scan the patient first in a transverse imaging plane. The CCA can be followed from its origin at the subclavian artery cephalad to the carotid bifurcation. Then, depending on the level of the bifurcation rela-

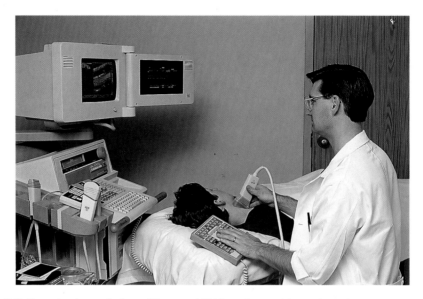

Fig. 3-7 Examination technique. The carotid bifurcation may be evaluated with the examiner sitting alongside or at the head of the patient, depending on individual preference. It is important that both the examiner and the patient are comfortable.

tive to the mandible, 3 to 4 cm of the proximal internal and external carotid arteries can be seen. A rapid transverse scan initially allows the examiner to plan the best approach for obtaining proper sagittal scan planes and to more easily follow the direction and course of the tortuous vessels. An initial assessment can also be made rapidly regarding the degree of stenosis.

DCI aids in the rapid identification of vessels since the flowing blood stands out from the gray-scale image. It is especially important to use optimal gain and flow sensitivity settings. The color gain should be adjusted so that color fills the entire vessel lumen without blending into the adjacent soft tissues. Frame rates vary inversely with the size of the area being displayed in color. Thus, the examiner must choose the optimal size of the color field depending on the expected clinical problem. To study a tortuous vessel a large field could be chosen, whereas to evaluate a possible occlusion a small field with a rapid pulse repetition rate should be chosen.

When using DCI, the flow of blood toward the head is usually displayed as red. Therefore, the CCA is colored red. Color in the jugular vein flows in the opposite direction and therefore appears blue. In normal patients, flow in the vertebral arteries is in the same direction as in the carotids (Fig. 3-3). To demonstrate flow in the transverse projection, the transducer must be angled generally cephalad so that the resulting transverse image is not a true indication of the same degree of stenosis that can be obtained with a transverse gray-scale image (in which the beam path should be perpendicular to the vessel wall). It is therefore important to scan both with and without color during the study. When possible, measurements of diameter and area stenosis should be made by

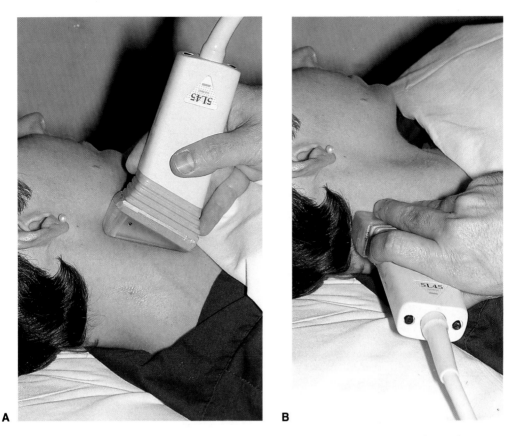

A   B

Fig. 3-8 Scanning approaches. Depending on the patient's anatomy, the carotid vessels may be evaluated by scanning either **(A)** anterior or **(B)** posterior to the sternocleidomastoid muscle. Often, both approaches are necessary for complete evaluation.

gray-scale imaging so that the transducer is perpendicular to the area being studied and a more accurate assessment may be made (Fig. 3-9).

Following examination in the transverse plane, the vessels are studied in a longitudinal plane. As with angiography, multiple longitudinal views are useful in fully evaluating the vessels. The CCA is scanned as far proximally as possible and is then followed distally to the bifurcation. Separate views of the CCA extending into the ICA and of the CCA extending into the ECA are then obtained. In most patients, it is difficult to obtain longitudinal views that simultaneously demonstrate the CCA, ICA, and ECA. An estimation of diameter stenosis can also be obtained from the longitudinal view.

The ECA can be identified by its branches

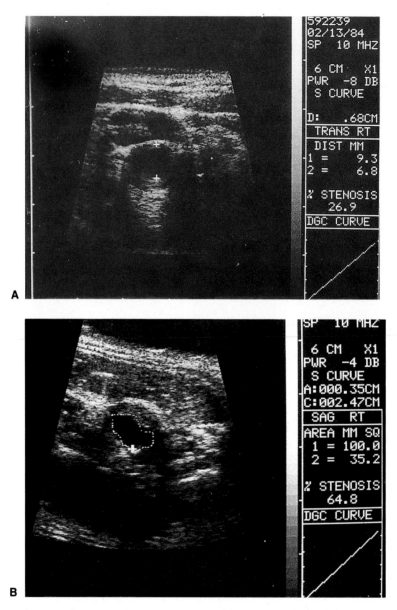

Fig. 3-9 Diameter measurements. **(A)** Vessel diameter stenosis is the ratio of the intima-to-intima measurement of the vessel lumen diameter to the residual lumen diameter measured at the site of greatest narrowing. **(B)** Area stenosis is the ratio of the vessel lumen area calculated from measurement of vessel circumference to the area of the residual lumen. Most reporting of carotid stenosis indicates estimated diameter reduction.

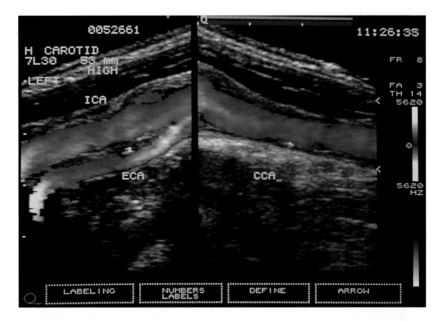

Fig. 3-10 Normal carotid vessels. Composite longitudinal scan using a posterior approach shows the common, external and internal carotid arteries. The ICA is the larger of the branches at the bifurcation and lies posterior and lateral to the ECA. This image was generated from two scans, and the apparent angulation of the distal CCA is a result of the need to reverse the orientation of the transducer for the two portions of the image. Note the normal flow reversal in the carotid bulb opposite the origin of the ECA.

(Fig. 3-5). It can also be identified, if necessary, by tapping on the temporal artery and noting changes in the Doppler spectrum. Usually the low resistance pattern of the Doppler spectrum of the ICA is sufficient to distinguish it from the high-resistance ECA. With DCI, throughout the cardiac cycle there is usually continuous color in the ICA, in contrast to intermittent color in the ECA. The ICA usually is larger and is located posterolateral to the ECA (Fig. 3-10). Usually several centimeters of the proximal ICA can be studied. Once the vessels are imaged transversely, a mental picture of the direction of the vessels allows the examiner to rapidly align the transducer to produce sagittal images quickly. Once the vessels have been imaged in color in this cursory manner, the examiner can look for areas of color saturation. The white areas within the color flow pattern

reflect areas of increased Doppler frequency shift. Although these areas represent sites of high Doppler frequency shifts, they do not always indicate abnormal elevations of systolic velocity. They do, however, direct the examiner to the sites where Doppler spectral analysis sampling and careful evaluation of plaque morphology should be made.

After the vessels have been imaged carefully and their flow patterns studied, pulsed-Doppler waveform analysis is performed from representative areas within the vessels to document blood flow velocities. Because the DCI image differentiates areas of normal and abnormal flow, it allows much more directed placement of the pulsed-Doppler sample volume. This markedly shortens examination times as compared with conventional duplex Doppler, in which the pulsed-Dopp-

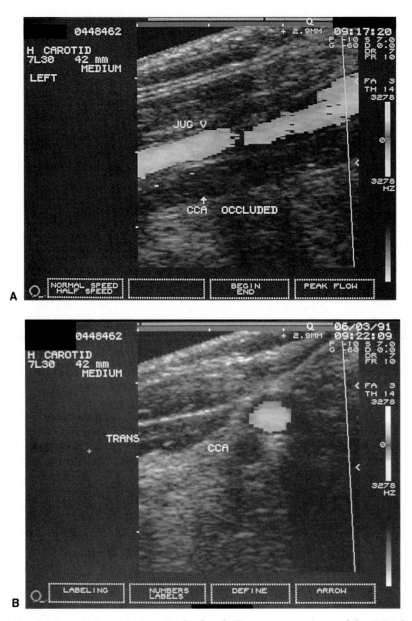

Fig. 3-11 CCA occlusion. **(A)** Longitudinal and **(B)** transverse views of the CCA by DCI show flow in the jugular vein (blue) but none in the CCA. Hypoechoic thrombus fills the lumen of the artery.

ler sample volume must be moved meticulously throughout the entire lumen of the vessel.

SPECIAL CONSIDERATIONS

Color is useful in directing attention to the sites where plaque is located. The plaque can then be studied to carefully characterize it into either homogeneous or heterogeneous patterns.[11] Characterization of plaque is best made by gray-scale imaging. Acute thrombosis may be sufficiently echogenic to be visualized by gray-scale imaging alone; however, hypoechoic or anechoic thrombus may be missed unless flow imaging is performed (Fig. 3-11).

After the vessels have been imaged carefully and the color flow patterns studied, pulsed-Doppler and Doppler spectrum waveform analysis are performed to measure increased blood flow velocities. This is done by moving a Doppler gate along the length of the imaged artery and sampling at discrete sites. The color patterns are used as a guide to determine the sites to be sampled since the color image shows the Doppler shift within each pixel.

We use a standardized Doppler examination to evaluate the carotid and vertebral arteries on the basis of spectral analysis. Measurements are made of the peak systolic and peak diastolic velocities in the CCA and ICA. The ratios of systolic and diastolic velocities in the ICA to those in the CCA are calculated. These four measurements are used to arrive at a determination of the degree of stenosis. These velocity measurements are most easily made from the sagittal scans (Fig. 3-12). DCI is helpful in ensuring that the Doppler angle is correctly chosen and that the velocity measurements are accurate since the direction of vessels can be followed more easily (Fig. 3-

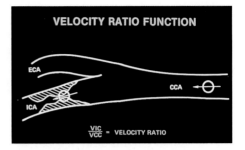

Fig. 3-12 Doppler measurements. Doppler measurements of the peak systolic and diastolic velocity are made at the site of greatest narrowing and in the CCA. The ratio of systolic and diastolic velocities in the ICA and CCA may be used to estimate the degree of stenosis in the ICA.

13). This produces more accurate velocity calculations.

If aliasing occurs, characteristic DCI changes appear (Fig. 3-2), and spectral waveforms appear clipped at the top (Fig. 3-14). To reduce alaising, one can (1) change the probe position to decrease the tissue path of the vessel, permitting a lower pulse repitition frequency; (2) increase the Doppler incidence angle; (3) use a lower-frequency Doppler; (4) add spectral components; or (5) use continuous-wave Doppler. Aliasing can occur in severe and critical stenoses, and it affects the measurement of systolic velocity to a much greater degree than that of diastolic velocity. When systolic spectral components are aliased to the extent that they cannot be measured accurately, peak end-diastolic velocity should be used to estimate stenosis.

The Doppler quantitative measure of stenosis is taken along with the direct measure of vessel narrowing to determine the degree of stenosis reported. If the degree of stenosis is small, the visual image may be more accurate than the Doppler data. The reverse is true for more significant stenosis. DCI aids in the determination of the residual lumen by providing contrast between the vessel wall and

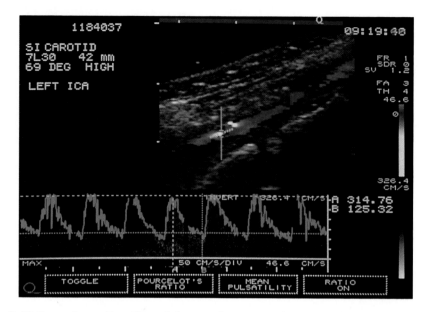

Fig. 3-13 Spectral sampling. One of the most important advantages of DCI is its ability to display flow from throughout the area of interest. This allows the selection of sampling sites for spectral Doppler and accurate estimation of the Doppler angle. This results in more accurate measurement of peak systolic and diastolic velocities. In this example the high-velocity jet associated with this 80 to 90 percent stenosis is quite small, and Doppler sampling without the use of DCI might have underestimated the Doppler changes.

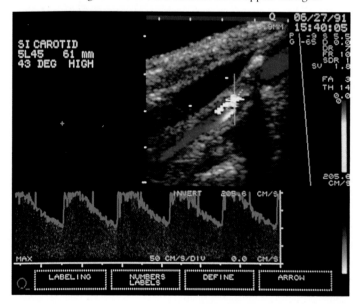

Fig. 3-14 Spectral Doppler aliasing. The high-frequency shift associated with this 70 to 80 percent stenosis of the internal carotid artery exceeds the Nyquist limit, and the highest frequencies are not displayed but appear as lower-frequency components beneath the baseline. (These are not shown in this image, but are typically displayed.)

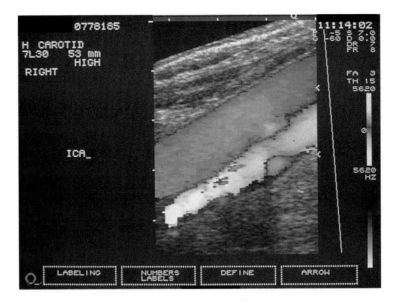

Fig. 3-15 Mild narrowing. Although quantitative assessment by spectral Doppler is essential to quantify stenoses of greater than 40 to 50 percent; it is less valuable in measurement of less severe stenosis. DCI, by providing contrast between the vessel wall and lumen, permits estimation of the effects of milder degrees of stenosis. Here stenosis of less than 40 percent, resulting from a small plaque on the deep wall of the vessel, is shown in the distal ICA.

the lumen, much as an intravascular contrast agent does in angiography (Fig. 3-15). In all cases, inspection and characterization of plaque and Doppler spectral analysis to quantitatively determine the degree of stenosis are equal parts of standard examination of the extracranial carotid vessels.

FLOW PATTERNS AND HEMODYNAMICS

In addition to the morphologic differences between the ICA and ECA, there are several hemodynamic differences that make these vessels distinguishable. The ICA supplies the brain parenchyma. Like other parenchymal organs (such as the liver, kidney, and testes), the brain has a low vascular resistance. Therefore, the pulsed-Doppler waveform from the ICA generally has a wide systolic peak and relatively high levels of diastolic

flow throughout the cardiac cycle (Fig. 3-16A). The ECA, on the other hand, supplies the facial muscles and the scalp. These tissues have a high vascular resistance, and for this reason the pulsed-Doppler waveform from the ECA has narrow systolic peaks and flow levels or complete absence of diastolic flow (Fig. 3-16B). These differing waveform characteristics can generally allow for rapid distinction between these two vessels. In problematic cases, one can tap the superficial temporal artery in front of the external auditory meatus and detect the transmitted pulsations from this external carotid branch within the external carotid waveform. Table 3-2 lists the anatomic and hemodynamic ways of distinguishing the ICA and ECA.

With more widespread use of DCI, attention has recently been turned toward the meaning and significance of flow patterns. In the past, glass models have been used to study flow

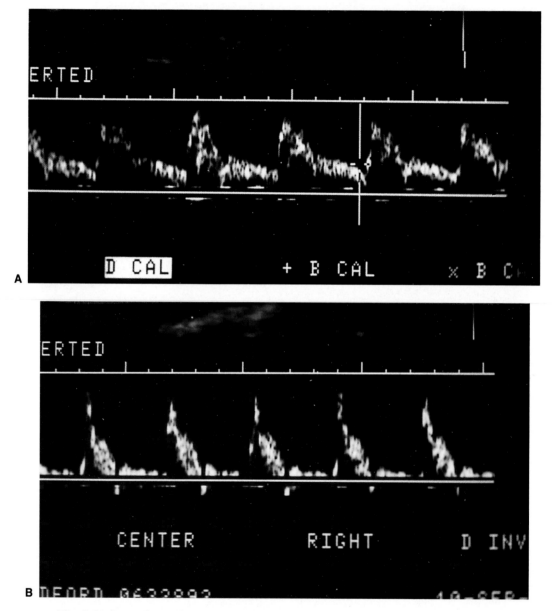

Fig. 3-16 Spectral waveforms. **(A)** The Doppler spectrum of the normal ICA is characterized by the presence of continuous flow through systole and diastole, reflecting the low resistance of the cerebral circulation supplied by the ICA. **(B)** The ECA waveform shows absent diastolic flow as it supplies a higher-resistance vascular bed.

Table 3-2 Differences in the Internal and
External Carotid Arteries

Characteristic	ICA	ECA
Size	Larger	Smaller
Location	Posterior and lateral	Anterior and medial
Branches	No	Yes
Waveform	Low resistance	High resistance
Temporal tap	No pulsations	Pulsations

in the carotid bifurcation.[12,13] These studies have predicted the presence of boundary layer separation and flow reversal in the carotid bulb. The energy of flowing blood can be divided into a static head (pressure) and a dynamic head (kinetic energy). At the bulb, the lumen of the vessel expands, resulting in a decrease in the average flow velocity and thus a decrease in the kinetic energy. To maintain total energy, pressure in this region increases. The increased pressure acts on the slowly moving blood at the peripheral aspect of the vessel lumen and causes localized flow reversal in this region. The region of flow reversal separates the normal boundary layer of slowly flowing blood away from the vessel wall and is therefore referred to as *boundary layer separation*. This flow reversal, which has been predicted experimentally, has now been identified routinely in vivo by using DCI (Fig. 3-6). Middleton et al. have documented that flow reversal was identified in essentially all (99 of 100) asymptomatic volunteers.[14] It is located in the peripheral aspect of the carotid bulb opposite the origin of the external carotid artery. The flow reversal appears in early or peak systole and persists into diastole for a variable period. During a portion of the diastolic phase of the cardiac cycle, the region of flow reversal is replaced by static blood. Distal to the bifurcation, the region of flow reversal migrates to the center of the ICA and extends from the superficial to the deep wall of the ICA. An analysis of these 100 bifurcations shows that the size, shape, and duration of flow reversal are extremely constant. At present, the exact significance of these variations is uncertain. It is interesting, however, that atherosclerotic plaque tends to originate and predominate precisely in the region of flow reversal. Long-term prospective studies are necessary to determine the significance of observed flow patterns in the ICA. However, it seems only logical that the unique information obtained from performing DCI at the carotid bifurcation indicates the individuals at greater risk for the development of localized atherosclerotic disease. In time, the role of DCI may extend well beyond that of identifying candidates for carotid endarterectomy or other interventional procedures. For the present, examiners should be aware of normal flow reversals, and their absence should prompt a careful search for subtle plaque.

In addition to showing gross changes such as flow reversal, DCI permits more subtle characteristics of laminar flow to be seen in the carotid vessels. The location of the high velocity jet stream of flow can usually be identified during systole (Fig. 3-17), and areas of slow flow and flow separation along the vessel wall are also shown (Fig. 3-18). Knowledge of these features of flow is helpful in selecting spectral sampling sites and in interpreting the spectral display.

PLAQUE CHARACTERIZATION

With the introduction of duplex scanners, examiners have become better able to investigate and try to understand the risks and causes of embolic stroke. It is well known that many patients with hemispheric symptoms have less than a 50 percent reduction in the diameter of their carotid vessels. It is theorized that in many of these patients the symptoms are caused by embolic episodes. It is thought that by differentiating different forms of plaque, a better understanding of who is at greater risk for embolic stroke will become apparent.

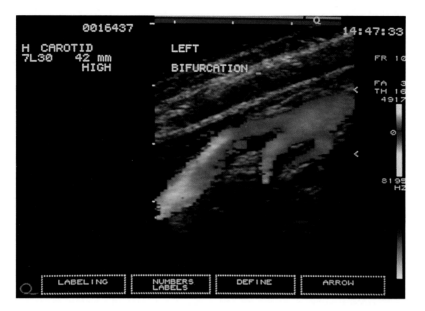

Fig. 3-17 Streamline flow. Higher velocities are displayed as less saturated colors in this image of the carotid bifurcation. Here the maximum velocities are not in the center of the vessel, as expected, but near the lateral wall of the vessel. Because flowing blood has inertia, the streamline typically drifts toward the outside wall of a curving vessel.

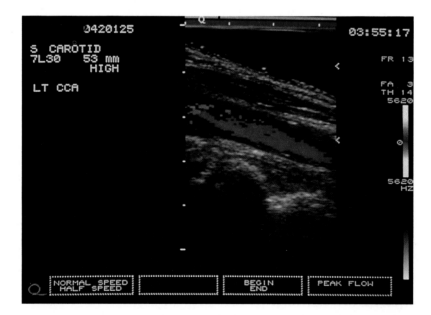

Fig. 3-18 Flow separation. This image is obtained in mid-diastole from the CCA. In diastole, average velocities are lower than in systole and forward flow continues only in the center of the vessel, with separation of flow from slowly moving or stationary blood along the vessel wall (dark areas).

Several vascular surgeons, including Imaparato et al.[15] and Lusby et al.,[16] have reported that the incidence of intraplaque hemorrhage in surgical specimens of carotid artery plaque from their symptomatic patients is significantly higher than that in specimens from asymptomatic patients. It is believed that embolization may result when intraplaque hemorrhage leads to intimal tears in the vessel lining, initiation of the clotting cascade, and thrombus formation over the tear. The resulting thrombus can then be incorporated into the vessel wall, resulting in increased stenosis, or can break off and embolize into distal vessels of the carotid circulation, leading to stroke.

With high-quality ultrasound imaging, it is now possible to evaluate the structure of plaque and the vessel wall and to detect intraplaque hemorrhage. Bluth et al.[11] have shown conclusively that intraplaque hemorrhage can be identified within the vessel wall with an accuracy of 90 percent, a sensitivity of 96 percent, and a specificity of 88 percent. Intraplaque hemorrhage and ulceration are found in plaque that presents a heterogeneous pattern. Plaques that are homogeneous in their sonographic appearance contain no pathologic evidence of intraplaque hemorrhage or ulceration. Others, including Reilly et al.[17] and O'Donnell et al.,[18] have shown similar findings.

Patients should be examined in the supine position with the head hyperextended and the neck either straight or oblique in the contralateral direction. Since the carotid vessels are relatively superficial, a high-frequency imaging probe (7.5 to 10 MHz) should be used to visualize vessel anatomy and vascular abnormalities optimally in both the transverse and sagittal planes. It is important to scan in both planes to properly assess the relationship of the plaque to the wall and not falsely identify a sonolucent space between the plaque and the wall caused by a position artifact.

Two different forms of plaque can be identified, homogeneous and heterogeneous.[11,17,19] Homogeneous plaque (Fig. 3-19) consists of plaque that is relatively uniform in texture compared with the soft tissues surrounding the vessel wall. Pathologically, this usually corresponds to dense laminated fibrous connective tissue. The surface of this plaque type is always smooth. Calcifications can be present in either form of plaque and do not enter into the scheme of classification.

Heterogeneous plaque (Fig. 3-20) has a complex echo pattern that contains at least one well-defined focal sonolucent area. This form of plaque contains areas of intraplaque hemorrhage. The intimal surface of this plaque can be smooth or irregular. When the surface is irregular, it is always heterogeneous. When the surface is smooth, it can be either homogeneous or heterogeneous, depending on the presence or absence of a focal sonolucent area within the plaque. Although all ulcerative plaques appear to be heterogeneous, not all heterogeneous plaques are ulcerated. There are no sonographic criteria to separate heterogeneous plaques that contain ulcerations from heterogeneous plaques that do not.[20] Perhaps with the advent of DCI some additional criteria may be developed.

Although it has been shown conclusively that we can sonographically identify intraplaque hemorrhage, the significance of this finding is still somewhat controversial. Sterpetti et al.[21] have shown in a prospective study that heterogeneous plaque is a significant risk factor for developing subsequent neurologic defects. In another study, Leahy et al.[22] showed that there was a significant increase in ipsilateral cerebral hemispheric symptoms in patients with heterogeneous plaque (50 percent with symptoms) over the incidence in patients with homogeneous plaque (22 percent with symptoms). However, additional long-term studies are needed to show conclusively that the presence of different forms of plaque

Fig. 3-19 Homogeneous plaque. **(A)** Artist's depiction of homogeneous plaque shows the uniform consistency of the fibrous tissue making up the plaque. **(B)** Ultrasound image of homogeneous plaque shows medium level echoes throughout the plaque. **(C & D)** Endarterectomy specimens of plaque characterized as homogeneous by ultrasound show fibrous tissue with no evidence of intraplaque hemorrhage. (Figs. A, C, and D from Bluth et al.,[11] with permission. Fig. B from Merritt and Bluth,[19] with permission.)

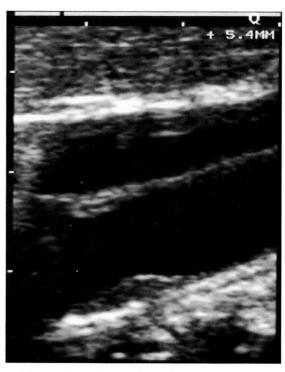

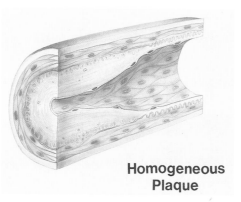

Homogeneous Plaque

A

B

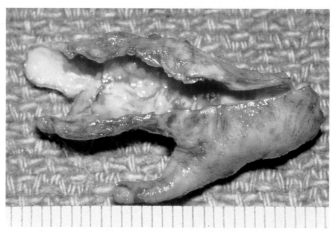

C

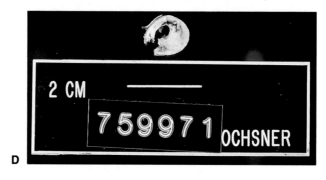

D

Fig. 3-20 Heterogeneous plaque. **(A)** Artist's depiction of heterogeneous plaque shows pools of lipid within the plaque, along with areas of intraplaque hemorrhage, and breakdown of the intima with spillage of plaque contents and hemorrhage into the vessel lumen. **(B)** Ultrasound image of heterogeneous plaque shows a large hypoechoic area (arrows) corresponding to intraplaque hemorrhage. **(C & D)** Endarterectomy specimens of plaque characterized as heterogeneous by ultrasound show large areas of hemorrhage (dark material). (Figs. A, C, and D from Bluth et al.,[11] with permission. Fig. B from Merritt and Bluth,[19] with permission.)

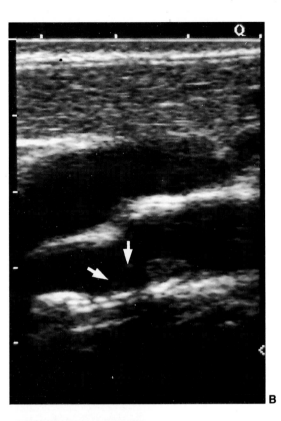

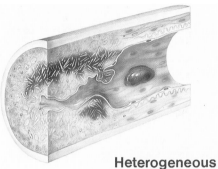

Heterogeneous
Plaque

A

B

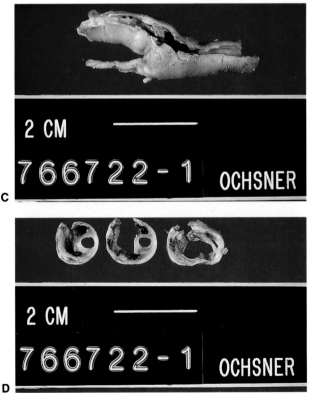

C

D

leads to a different incidence of neurologic symptoms and stroke before the concept of treating patients differently on the basis of plaque characterization becomes uniformly accepted. Nevertheless, it is important at present to appreciate the differences in plaque features and to categorize plaque whenever possible into these two groupings so that they can be monitored for change. For now, it would seem logical to monitor patients with potentially unstable heterogeneous plaque more closely than patients with homogeneous plaque.

DOPPLER EVALUATION

The Doppler portion of the duplex examination is complementary to imaging and is used to assess luminal narrowing and to determine the presence and degree of flow restriction. In the past, flow restriction has been assessed by angiography and digital vascular imaging (DVI). Now, with better Doppler instrumentation and more sophisticated data analysis, sensitivities and specificities ranging from 84 to 99 percent and 90 to 95 percent accuracy, respectively, with duplex Doppler as compared with angiography have been reported for the assessment of the carotid bifurcation stenosis.[1,2,3,4,23-34] As a result, duplex Doppler and DCI evaluation of the carotid arteries are increasingly being used as the primary means of evaluating for carotid disease. DCI provides several enhancements to conventional duplex Doppler in the evaluation of the extracranial carotid system (Table 3-3).

Initially, Doppler analysis was performed by using frequency data. Now it is more common to use velocity calculations. This is because frequency data are more difficult to obtain and compare, as they depend on both the incident Doppler frequency and the Doppler angle. With velocity calculations, angle correction occurs and is accurate as long as the incident angle does not approach

Table 3-3 Contributions of DCI to Cerebrovascular Evaluation

Global Doppler sampling
Simultaneous real-time display of flow and vessel wall
Improved contrast between vessel wall and lumen
Improved estimation of residual lumen
Improved visualization of plaque
Identification of turbulence and high velocity jets
More accurate measurement of Doppler angle
Reduced examination time
Greater diagnostic confidence

70 degrees. Also, velocity measurements are independent of the transmission frequency of the Doppler transducer.[1] With the use of velocity data, information from different machines and different laboratories can be compared, allowing better follow-up of patients.

Although the point is still somewhat controversial, most agree that surgery to alleviate flow-limiting stenosis is appropriate only when there was a 70 percent or greater area of reduction in the ICA lumen.[35] Therefore, it is of great value to be able to separate the different grades of carotid stenosis. Five quantitative Doppler measurements are used to accurately assess flow-limiting stenosis:

Peak systolic velocity (PSV) is determined at the point of maximum stenosis. The peak velocity (cm/s) is measured at the peak systolic point of the cardiac cycle.

Peak end-diastolic velocity (PEDV) is determined at the point of maximum stenosis. The peak diastolic velocity (cm/s) is measured at the endpoint of the cardiac cycle and is the peak velocity at end diastole.

Peak systolic velocity ratio (SVR) is the peak velocity at the point of maximum stenosis in the ICA (V_{ICA}) divided by the peak velocity in the unobstructed CCA (V_{CCA}) 2 cm or more below the bifurcation (SVR $= V_{ICA}/V_{CCA}$).

Peak diastolic velocity ratio (DVR) is the peak diastolic velocity at the point of maximum

Table 3-4 Doppler Criteria for Vessel Narrowing

Category	Percent Stenosis[a]	Peak Systolic Velocity (cm/s)	Peak Diastolic Velocity (cm/s)	Peak Systolic Velocity Ratio	Peak Diastolic Velocity Ratio	Spectral Broadening (cm/s)
Normal	0	<110	<40	<1.8	<2.4	<30
Mild	1–39	<110	<40	<1.8	<2.4	<40
Moderate	40–59	<130	<40	<1.8	<2.4	<40
Severe	60–79	>130	>40	>1.8	>2.4	>40
Critical	80–99	>250	>100	>3.7	>5.5	>80

[a] Diameter stenosis.
(From Bluth et al.,[1] with permission.)

stenosis in the ICA divided by the peak diastolic velocity in the unobstructed CCA 1 cm or more below the bifurcation (DVR $= V_{ICA}/V_{CCA}$).

Spectral broadening—turbulence results in an increased range (distribution) of flow velocities. Spectral broadening should be determined distal to the stenosis and is usually measured at peak systole. It can be quantitated by measuring the range of velocities at the 50 percent amplitude level of the Doppler power spectrum.

When the quantitative Doppler assessment has been made, the values obtained can be compared with standard tables (Table 3-4) to determine the degree of stenosis.[1] Although one may estimate the degree of stenosis from the DCI image, accurate estimation is possible only when using Doppler spectral analysis and identifying velocity changes (Fig. 3-21).

It should be noted that measurements of systolic and diastolic velocity or velocity ratios do not permit highly accurate quantification of narrowing that is less than 50 to 60 percent. Above this level, the degree of stenosis should be quantified by using peak velocities and velocity ratios. Use of the diastolic velocity ratio is recommended in estimating diameter stenosis greater than 80 percent.[1] Use

of the systolic and diastolic velocity ratios is particularly important in patients who have significant cardiovascular problems such as hypertension, severe bradycardia, and cardiac output failure. For example, a hypertensive patient with normal carotid vessels may have a significantly elevated peak systolic velocity. However, the systolic velocity ratio should be normal because of equally elevated peak systolic velocity in the common carotid artery. In some patients, particularly those with arrhythmias, aberrant carotid waveforms invalidate Doppler spectral analysis data.

In general, velocities in the CCA should be symmetric. When they are not and there is no technical error of angulation, the asymmetry could be the result of a severe contralateral ICA stenosis or occlusion or a severe ipsilateral proximal CCA stenosis. Special attention should be given to assessment of these situations.

DCI and Doppler assessments of the degree of stenosis usually agree. When there is disagreement, greater reliance should be placed on image assessment when the spectral Doppler measurements suggest less than a 50 to 60 percent stenosis. Greater reliance should be placed on the Doppler assessment when the degree of stenosis by Doppler

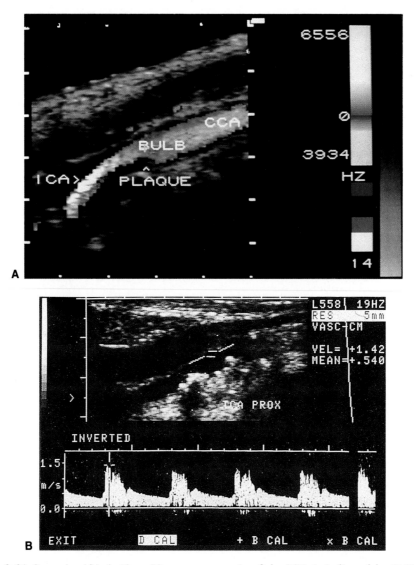

Fig. 3-21 Stenosis. **(A)** A 40 to 50 percent stenosis of the ICA is indicated by DCI; the estimation of stenosis is based on the imaging findings. **(B)** The spectral Doppler measurements from the same vessel are shown. These values are also consistent with 40 to 50 percent stenosis. (*Figure continues.*)

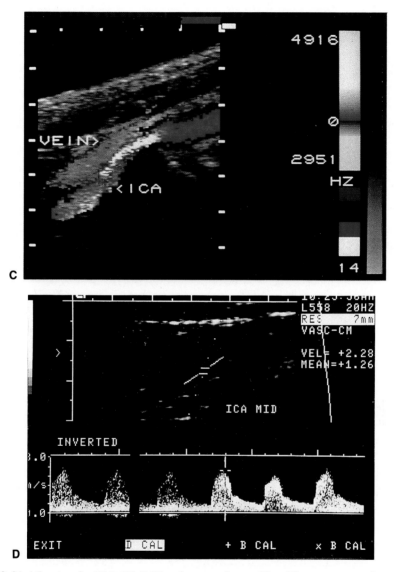

Fig. 3-21 (*Continued*). **(C & D)** DCI and spectra from a 70 to 80 percent stenosis are shown. (*Figure continues.*)

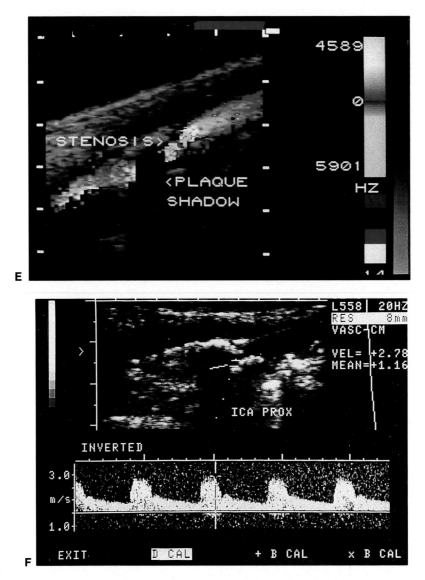

Fig. 3-21 (*Continued*). (**E & F**) The stenosis is 80 to 90 percent. Although DCI is used to identify the area of narrowing, velocity measurements made by spectral Doppler are always performed to grade the stenosis.

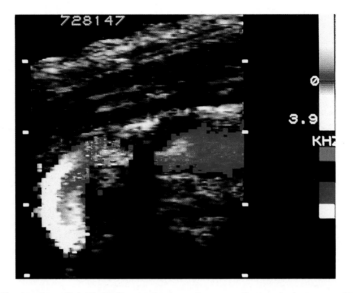

Fig. 3-22 Shadowing. Calcified plaque obscures the area of stenosis; however, DCI permits identification of the high-velocity jet as it emerges from the shadow of the plaque and provides guidance for spectral Doppler sampling. In this case the velocities were not indicative of a hemodynamically significant lesion.

criteria is greater than 50 to 60 percent stenosis (i.e., systolic velocity ratio of >1.8). In addition, when there is a disagreement between image Doppler assessment, the examiner should first be careful to ensure that the correct angle is being used (45 to 60 degrees). With DCI, the residual lumen generally can easily be seen in patients with significant stenosis unless there is extensive calcification. As a result, patients who have extremely high stenosis (greater than 95 percent), and therefore have velocities reduced to normal levels, can be more easily identified. In tortuous vessels, or vessels in which there is extensive calcification, uncertainty in determining the true angle may make velocity readings unreliable. DCI is useful in helping to eliminate some of these pitfalls by identifying the true course of the vessel and allowing proper interrogation of the vessel. For example, if calcified plaque obscures the area of stenosis from view, DCI may permit identification of the high-velocity jet as it emerges from the area of calcification and allow precise placement of the spectral sample volume for velocity measurement (Fig. 3-22).

DCI has been particularly valuable in accurately identifying ICA occlusion and detecting preocclusive high-grade stenosis. When maximum flow sensitivity settings are used, no evidence of flow is noted in the occluded vessel. In addition, a characteristic flow reversal is seen just proximal to the site of the occlusion (Fig. 3-23). In both situations, damping of flow in the ipsilateral CCA is noted. This is characterized by decreased, absent, or even reversed end-diastolic flow. DCI is also an excellent method for showing collateral flow in the ECA after CCA occlusion (Fig. 3-24).[36] Several recent articles[5,6,37] report a greater than 95 percent accuracy in identifying carotid artery occlusion by using

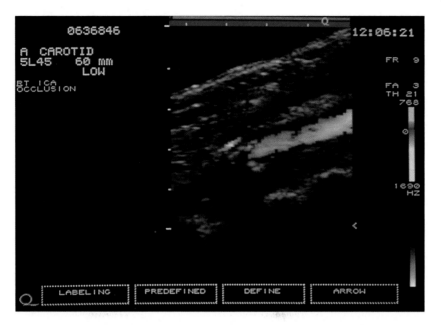

Fig. 3-23 Carotid occlusion. DCI reveals abrupt termination of flow in the carotid artery. There is reversal of flow (blue) at the occluded stump of the vessel, a common finding in complete obstruction.

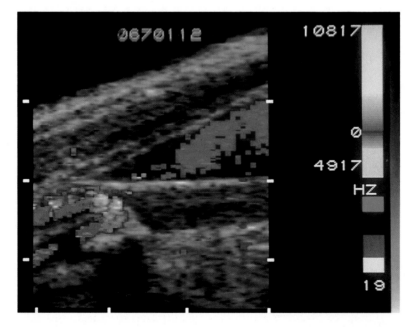

Fig. 3-24 Collateral flow. Reversed flow in the ECA (blue vessel on left) is shown in a patient with CCA occlusion. The ICA (red vessel on left) is supplied by retrograde flow in the ECA and shows flow in a normal direction. (From Merritt,[36] with permission.)

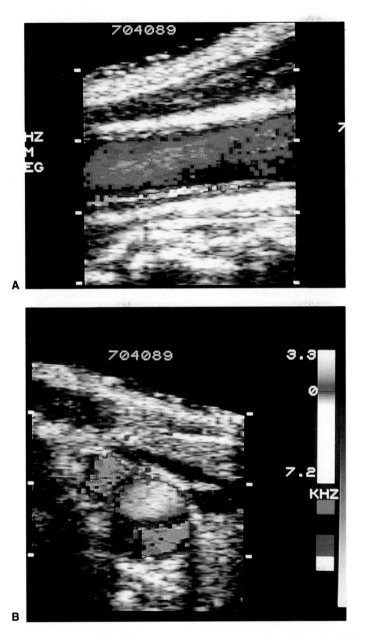

Fig. 3-25 Dissection. Dissection of the CCA is shown in **(A)** longitudinal and **(B)** transverse images. The true lumen (red) shows flow toward the brain, while the false lumen (blue) exhibits reversed flow, presumably as a result of differences in the pressure gradients in the true and false lumens. (From Merritt,[9] with permission.)

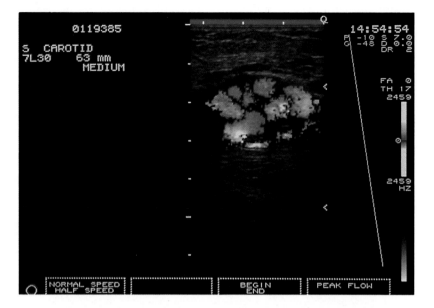

Fig. 3-26 Carotid body tumor. DCI of a mass at the carotid bifurcation reveals a hypervascular tumor. The adjacent carotid arteries and jugular vein were normal.

DCI and spectral analysis. DCI is also useful in identifying unusual abnormalities such as carotid artery dissections[38] (Fig. 3-25) and carotid body tumors (Fig. 3-26) and in distinguishing carotid aneurysms from tortuous vessels.

POSTENDARTERECTOMY FOLLOW-UP

The follow-up of patients after endarterectomy is a useful application of duplex sonography (Fig. 3-27).[39–41] Since it is noninvasive, has virtually no morbidity, and is relatively inexpensive and highly accurate, it is gaining wide acceptance by both clinicians and patients. The exact incidence of restenosis following endarterectomy varies in the literature between 1 and 36 percent.[41] The timing of restenosis varies depending on the etiology. Palmaz et al.[42] reported that neointimal fibromuscular hyperplasia is the cause

of restenosis when it occurs within 2 years of carotid endarterectomy. Technical factors such as incomplete removal of the distal extent of the plaque or vascular clamp damage reportedly can lead to a disturbance in laminar flow and may enhance neointimal hyperplasia. After 2 years, when restenosis occurs, the etiology most commonly is atherosclerosis. We have observed some unusual DCI flow patterns and elevated velocity measurements in patients who have undergone vein patch bypass procedures. Additional studies of the long-term outcome are needed to determine the exact significance of these unusual findings.

VERTEBRAL ARTERIES

The vertebral arteries can generally be visualized during study of the carotid arteries. DCI adds to this rapid identification. The vertebral arteries are frequently visualized on transverse scans during an examination of the

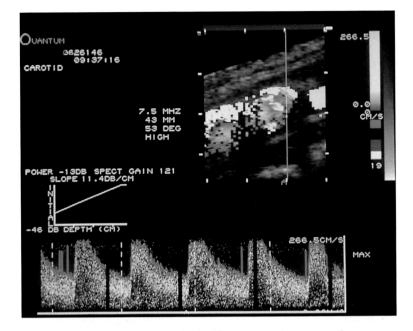

Fig. 3-27 Endarterectomy restenosis. A significant stenosis at an endarterectomy site is shown in a patient 3 years after endarterectomy. In this case an intimal flap, undetected at the time of surgery, probably contributed to the poor result shown.

carotid arteries (Fig. 3-3). They are best visualized in the sagittal projection by continuing to turn the transducer obliquely beyond the CCA. They are identified between the spinous processes of the cervical spine (Fig. 3-28A) and are thereby distinguished from the ascending cervical branch of the thyrocervical trunk. As a result, the complete vessel cannot be imaged. Parts of the vertebral arteries can be visualized by sonography in more than 80 percent of cases.[8,43,44] At times, spectral analysis is required to distinguish the vertebral vein from the vertebral artery (Fig. 3-28B). The vein runs parallel to the artery and is particularly difficult to identify when the vertebral artery is occluded, congenitally absent, or dysplastic.

Identification of vertebral stenosis is very difficult. Visonà et al.[44] determined that a peak systolic flow greater than 2 KHz (with a Doppler angle of between 45 and 70 degrees) indicates a 50 to 90 percent stenosis. However, since much of the vertebral arteries cannot be visualized, including frequently the origin, it is very difficult to identify stenosis. There are no universally accepted criteria for recognizing vertebral artery stenosis.

Subclavian steal syndrome, however, is far easier to identify than vertebral stenosis. In this syndrome, a stenosis or occlusion of the proximal subclavian artery results in reversal of the flow of blood. Blood flows from the basilar circulation, via the vertebral artery, to supply the ischemic arm. As a result, the diagnosis is made by identifying reversed flow in the vertebral arteries (Fig. 3-29). These arteries can be visualized in more than 80 percent of patients, and, with DCI, the direction of blood flow can be identified rapidly and accurately.

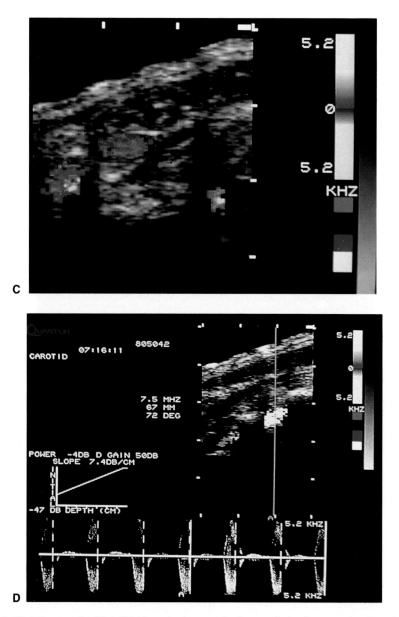

Fig. 3-29 (*Continued*). (**C & D**) Flow in the vertebral artery is in the opposite direction from that in the CCA and in the same direction as in the jugular vein. This indicates reversal of vertebral flow and is seen in the subclavian steal syndrome.

SUMMARY

Duplex sonography and DCI have now become standard modalities for imaging of the extracranial carotid and vertebral arteries. They are equivalent in accuracy to arteriography in the evaluation of flow-limiting stenosis. In addition, the newest scanners all appear to have high-resolution imaging systems capable of characterizing plaque properly. DCI currently leads to more rapid scanning and greater ease in evaluating more difficult patients. The most important advance with DCI will come in the future, when there is better understanding of the significance of the Doppler color-flow patterns now being observed. At present, duplex sonography and DCI remain the only imaging modalities that can evaluate the complete spectrum of abnormalities of the extracranial carotid and vertebral vessels, from minimal stenosis to complete occlusion. As a result, they are valuable tools in the diagnosis of disease.

REFERENCES

1. Bluth EI, Stavros AT, Marich KW, et al: Carotid duplex sonography: a multi-center recommendation for standardized imaging and Doppler criteria. RadioGraphics 8:487, 1988
2. Jacobs NM, Grant EG, Schellinger D, et al: Duplex carotid sonography: criteria for stenosis, accuracy, and pitfalls. Radiology 154:385, 1985
3. Langlois Y, Roedeter GO, Chan A, et al: Evaluating carotid artery disease; the concordance between pulsed Doppler spectrum analysis and angiography. Ultrasound Med Biol 9:51, 1983
4. Steinke W, Kloetzsch C, Hennerici M: Carotid artery disease assessed by color Doppler flow imaging: correlation with standard Doppler sonography and angiography. AJNR 11:259, 1990
5. Erickson SJ, Mewissen MW, Foley WD, et al: Stenosis of the internal carotid artery: assessment using color Doppler imaging compared with angiography. AJR 152:1299, 1989
6. Polak JF, Dobkin GR, O'Leary DH, et al: Internal carotid artery stenosis: accuracy and reproducibility of color-Doppler-assisted duplex imaging. Radiology 173:793, 1989
7. Hallam MJ, Reid JM, Cooperberg PL: Color-flow Doppler and conventional duplex scanning of the carotid bifurcation: prospective, double-blind, correlative study. AJR 152:1101, 1989
8. Bluth EI, Merritt CRB, Sullivan MA, et al: Usefulness of duplex ultrasound in evaluating vertebral arteries. J Ultrasound Med 8:229, 1989
9. Merritt CRB: Doppler color flow imaging. J Clin Ultrasound 15:591, 1987
10. Grant EG, Wong W, Tessler F, Perrella R: Cerebrovascular ultrasound imaging. Radiol Clin North Am 26:1111, 1988
11. Bluth EI, Kay D, Merritt CRB, et al: Sonographic characterization of carotid plaque—detection of hemorrhage. AJR 146:1061, 1986
12. Lo Gerfo FW, Nowak MD, Quist WC: Structural details of boundary layer separation in a model human carotid bifurcation under steady and pulsatile flow conditions. J Vasc Surg 2:263, 1985
13. Zarins CK, Giddens DP, Bharadvaj BK, et al: Carotid bifurcation atherosclerosis: quantitative correlation of plaque localization with flow velocity profiles and wall shear stress. Circ Res 53:502, 1983
14. Middleton W, Foley W, Lawson T: Flow reversal in the normal carotid bifurcation: color Doppler flow imaging analysis. Radiology 167:207, 1988
15. Imparato AM, Riles TS, Mintzer R, Baumann FG: The importance of hemorrhage in the relationship between gross morphologic characteristics and cerebral symptoms in 376 carotid artery plaques. Ann Surgery 197:195, 1983
16. Lusby RJ, Ferrell LD, Ehrenfeld WK, et al: Carotid plaque hemorrhage: its role in production of cerebral ischemia. Arch Surg 117:1479, 1982
17. Reilly LM, Lusby RJ, Hughes L, et al: Carotid plaque histology using real-time ultrasonography. Clinical and therapeutic implications. Am J Surg 146:188, 1983
18. O'Donnell TF Jr, Erodes L, Mackey WC, et al: Correlation of B-mode ultrasound imaging and arteriography with pathologic find-

ings at carotid endarterectomy. Arch Surg 120:443, 1985

19. Merritt CRB, Bluth EI: Ultrasonographic characterization of carotid plaque. In Labs KH (ed): Diagnostic Vascular Ultrasound. Hodder & Stoughton, London (in press)

20. Bluth EI, McVay L, Merritt CRB, Sullivan MA: The identification of ulcerative plaque with high resolution duplex carotid scanning. J Ultrasound Med 1:73, 1988

21. Sterpetti AV, Schultz RD, Feldhaus RJ, et al: Ultrasonographic features of carotid plaque and the risk of subsequent neurologic defects. Surgery 104:652, 1988

22. Leahy AL, McCollum PT, Feeley TM, et al: Duplex ultrasonography and selection of patients for carotid endarterectomy: plaque morphology or luminal narrowing? J Vasc Surg 8:558, 1988

23. Robinson ML, Sacks D, Perlmutter GS, Marinelli DL: Diagnostic criteria for carotid duplex sonography. AJR 151:1045, 1988

24. Garth KE, Carroll BA, Sommer FG, Oppenheimer DA: Duplex ultrasound scanning of the carotid arteries with velocity spectrum analysis. Radiology 147:823, 1983

25. Jackson VP, Kuehn DS, Bendick PJ, et al: Duplex carotid sonography: correlation with digital subtraction angiography and conventional angiography. J Ultrasound Med 4:239, 1985

26. Fell G, Phillips DJ, Chikos PM, et al: Ultrasonic duplex scanning for disease of the carotid artery. Circulation 64:1191, 1981

27. Blackshear WM Jr, Phillips DJ, Chikos PM, et al: Carotid artery velocity patterns in normal and stenotic vessels. Stroke 11:67, 1980

28. Keagy BA, Pharr WF, Thomas D, Bowles DE: Evaluation of the peak frequency ratio (PFR) measurement in the detection of internal carotid artery stenosis. J Clin Ultrasound 10:109, 1982

29. Friedman SG, Hainline B, Feinberg AW, et al: Use of diastolic velocity ratios to predict significant carotid artery stenosis. Stroke 19:910, 1988

30. Dreisbach JN, Seibert CE, Smazal SF, et al: Duplex sonography in the evaluation of carotid artery disease. AJNR 4:678, 1983

31. Vaisman U, Wojciechowski M: Carotid artery disease: new criteria for evaluation by sonographic duplex scanning. Radiology 158:253, 1986

32. Kotval PS: Doppler waveform parvus and tardus. A sign of proximal flow obstruction. J Ultrasound Med 8:435, 1989

33. Withers CE, Gosink BB, Keightley AM, et al: Duplex carotid sonography. Peak systolic velocity in quantifying internal carotid artery stenosis. J Ultrasound Med 9:345, 1990

34. Taylor DC, Strandness DE Jr: Carotid artery duplex scanning. J Clin Ultrasound 15:635, 1987

35. Matcher DB, Goldstein LB, Oddone EZ, et al: Carotid Endarterectomy. A Review of the Literature Regarding Risks and Complications. RAND Corp, Santa Monica, CA, 1992

36. Merritt CRB: Duplex and color Doppler in the evaluation of the extracranial carotid arteries. In Labs KH (ed): Diagnostic Vascular Ultrasound. Hodder & Stoughton, London (in press)

37. Middleton WD, Foley WD, Lawson TL: Color-flow Doppler imaging of carotid artery abnormalities. AJR 150:419, 1988

38. Bluth EI, Shyn PB, Sullivan MA, Merritt CRB: Doppler color flow imaging of carotid artery dissection. J Ultrasound Med 8:149, 1988

39. Glover JL, Bendick PJ, Dilley RS, et al: Restenosis following carotid endarterectomy: evaluation by duplex ultrasonography. Arch Surg 120:678, 1985

40. Aldoori MI, Baird RN: Prospective assessment of carotid endarterectomy by clinical and ultrasonic methods. Br J Surg 74:926, 1987

41. Pelz D, Rankin RN, Ferguson G: Intravenous digital subtraction angiography and duplex ultrasonography in postoperative assessment of carotid endarterectomy. J Neorosurg 66:88, 1987

42. Palmaz JC, Hunter G, Carson SN, French SW: Postoperative carotid restenosis due to neointimal fibromuscular hyperplasia. Radiology 148:699, 1983

43. Davis PC, Nilsen B, Braun IF, Hoffman JC Jr: A prospective comparison of duplex sonography vs angiography of the vertebral arteries. AJNR 7:1059, 1986

44. Visonà A, Lusiani L, Castellani V, et al: The echo-Doppler (duplex) system for the detection of vertebral artery occlusive disease: comparison with angiography. J Ultrasound Med 5:247, 1986

4

Peripheral Arteries

John S. Pellerito
Kenneth J. W. Taylor

During the past decade there has been an increasing trend away from invasive imaging techniques such as angiography. Although contrast angiography is still widely regarded as the gold standard for the assessment of vascular disease, it has several notable limitations, the most important being that it provides an anatomic depiction of a functional deficit, and the two are often not well related. The vascular surgeon needs to know whether there is sufficient perfusion of the limb to maintain viability and adequate flow to the muscles during various degrees of exercise. This is most clearly related to the pressure gradient across any stenosis rather than to estimates of luminal reduction, with their very well-recognized inter- and intra-observer variations. Segmental blood pressures are of some value in assessing pressure gradients across a stenosis, but pull-through pressure measurements at angiography produce the most accurate measurements of pressure gradient. The clinician also needs a technique that is noninvasive and can be repeated on many subsequent occasions to monitor the natural history of the disease and the need for intervention. The use of noninvasive Doppler color imaging (DCI) in-

stead of repeated contrast angiography for the diagnosis and surveillance of vascular pathology is therefore a major advance in diagnostic imaging.

The introduction of duplex Doppler to peripheral vascular evaluation adds a very useful modality that allows assessment of severity of disease. Duplex Doppler ultrasonography is also an examination that is easily repeated, so it allows longitudinal assessment of worsening peripheral vascular disease, graft patency, or both. Peak systolic velocity measurement and waveform characterization are the primary parameters for disease localization since the peak velocities produced at a focal stenosis correlate to a first approximation with the pressure gradient across it (the kinetic energy imparted to the red blood cells is derived from the static energy of the pressure gradient). Furthermore, the Doppler waveforms indicate the presence or absence of disease. For example, a normal triphasic waveform in the popliteal artery usually excludes the presence of surgically significant disease in the proximal aortic, iliac, and femoral segments. However, Doppler waveforms have some limitations:

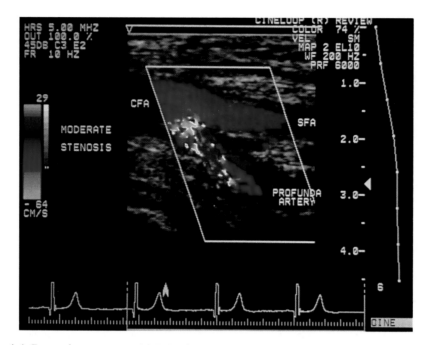

Fig. 4-1 Femoral artery stenosis. DCI demonstrates a focal color change due to aliasing in a stenosis at the origin of the profunda femoral artery.

they do not differentiate proximal from distal disease well; furthermore, pulsed Doppler shows the hemodynamic state at a single point only, requiring a time-consuming examination of the entire vessel.

DCI examination greatly facilitates evaluation of an entire arterial segment and allows a rapid overview to disclose any focal stenotic areas for interrogation by pulsed Doppler and quantitation of peak velocity (Fig. 4-1). It allows estimation of the length of the flow disturbance and the recognition of the presence of multiple focal stenoses. DCI is therefore extremely important for peripheral vascular evaluation. However, it must be stressed that DCI should not be used alone as a noninvasive angiogram that merely shows the anatomy of the vessel lumen, but should be combined with pulsed Doppler to quantitate the severity of the stenosis by the estimation of peak velocity and demonstration of poststenotic turbulence.

NORMAL LOWER LIMB ARTERIAL EVALUATION

The normal lower limb vascular examination should start at the aorta and extend distally to the dorsalis pedis. Ideally, the patient should be fasting, although this may not always be possible. With the patient lying supine, DCI and pulsed Doppler are used in a complementary fashion to demonstrate the size of the abdominal aorta and the presence of normal flow in the aorta, common iliac artery, and external iliac artery. For quantitative assessment, pulsed Doppler is used. The sample volume should be placed in the center of the vessel lumen and recordings obtained at a Doppler angle of 60 degrees or less. Waveforms obtained from the upper aorta should show a clear window under the time–velocity waveform, indicating the presence of plug flow (Fig. 4-2). In the lower aorta, a reversed component should be pres-

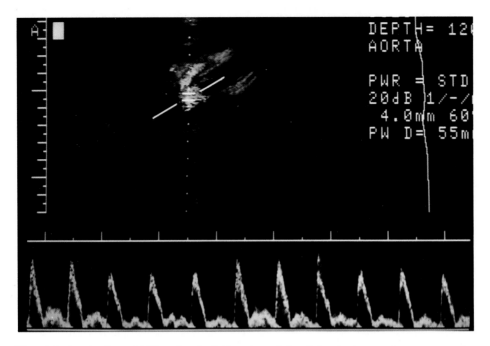

Fig. 4-2 Aortic flow. DCI and pulsed Doppler of the abdominal aorta demonstrate plug flow characterized by a clear window under the spectral envelope in systole.

ent converting the lower aortic waveform into the typical normal triphasic form of the healthy vessel.

The aorta usually divides at the level of the umbilicus. By scanning slightly obliquely, both common iliac arteries can be seen by DCI in the majority of patients. When possible, these arteries should be traced into the external iliac arteries and waveforms demonstrating the typical triphasic response should be elicited from each vessel (Fig. 4-3). Forward flow is seen in systole, followed by a brief reverse-flow component early in diastole. A third, forward-flow component is seen in late diastole; this component may be absent in noncompliant, atherosclerotic vessels. The reverse-flow component is a reflection of the high distal peripheral vascular resistance. This may be abolished by the presence of a significant stenosis or by vasodilatation due to exercise or reactive hyper-

emia (Fig. 4-4). In some patients, gas in the colon and small bowel prevents effective display of the iliac vessels. These limitations are particularly marked in very obese patients, in whom extensive scattering by subcutaneous and omental fat seriously interferes with ultrasonic visualization. Particular effort should be made to examine the aortoiliac segments when an abnormality of the proximal common femoral waveform is discovered. Limitations of ultrasonic access do not apply to the lower limb vessels from the level of the inguinal ligament down. Since these arteries are relatively superficial, transducers in the 5- to 10-MHz range with a Doppler frequency of 5 MHz can be used.

The external iliac artery becomes the femoral artery as it passes deep to the inguinal ligament, and at this point it is found midway between the anterior superior iliac spine and the pubic tubercle. Palpation in this position

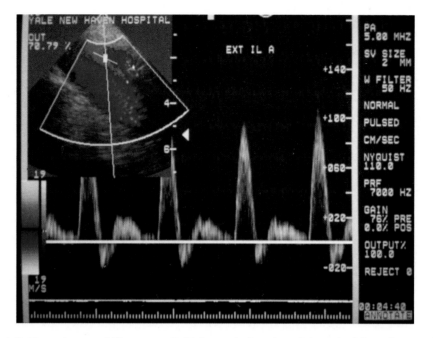

Fig. 4-3 Normal external iliac artery. DCI shows the location of the pulsed-Doppler sample volume within the external iliac artery. Pulsed Doppler demonstrates a triphasic waveform with a narrow systolic window representing red blood cells moving at the same velocity.

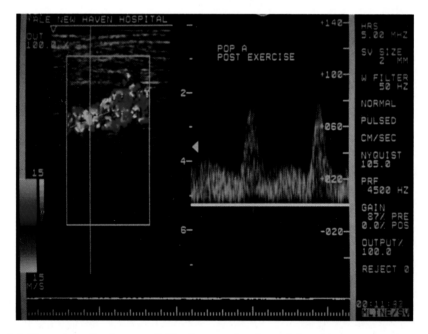

Fig. 4-4 Normal popliteal artery. Following exercise, loss of diastolic reversal and spectral broadening result from peripheral vasodilatation.

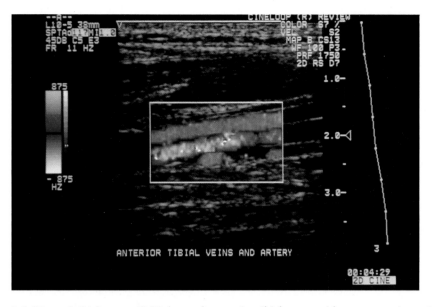

Fig. 4-5 Normal tibial artery. DCI shows the anterior tibial artery with accompanying paired veins.

immediately discloses the position of the artery. The linear array transducer is aligned longitudinally with the common femoral artery, and the normal triphasic waveform is elicited from the proximal artery. This process is repeated down the leg to demonstrate the bifurcation of the common femoral artery into the superficial and profunda femoral vessels. It should be recalled that bifurcations show a predilection for the development of arteriosclerosis, and special attention should be paid to these areas. The superficial femoral artery is traced down the leg into Hunter's canal. The most difficult part of the artery to demonstrate is usually that in Hunter's canal, because the vessel courses posteriorly towards the popliteal fossa, especially when the leg is large. This is also an area at high risk for arteriosclerosis and is a common site for focal stenoses. It is therefore extremely important to assess this area and obtain a normal waveform from it.

The popliteal vessels are best examined with the patient prone, although for less mobile patients a decubitus position suffices. For the immobile, the leg can be rotated laterally or lifted and the transducer placed under the leg in the popliteal fossa. Again, a normal triphasic waveform should be elicited, and at the lower extent of the popliteal artery the normal trifurcation is visualized.

Before the development of sensitive color Doppler, demonstrating the entire length of the anterior and posterior tibial and peroneal arteries was challenging and time-consuming. Distal examination was usually limited to analysis of the waveforms obtained from the vessels around the ankle. It is now possible to display color flow throughout the small vessels of the lower limb (Fig. 4-5).

QUANTITATION OF PERIPHERAL VASCULAR DISEASE

The quantitation of peripheral vascular disease in most laboratories still relies on criteria derived from the pulsed-Doppler waveforms.[1] Minimal disease, usually defined as

0 to 19 percent luminal reduction, consists of mild spectral broadening causing partial filling in of the normal window under the time–velocity waveform. The triphasic waveform is preserved, and the peak velocities can increase up to 30 percent more than in the prior segment. The next category is usually defined as 20 to 49 percent luminal diameter reduction. Again, there is spectral broadening, but in addition, the velocities increase up to double those in the proximal segment. The reverse-flow component is retained in diastole. Neither category constitutes surgically significant disease.

Surgically significant disease falls into a single large category of 50 to 99 percent diameter reduction, although the severity of stenosis within this range can be stratified to some extent on the basis of the Doppler changes. The findings of surgically significant disease consist of an increase in the peak systolic velocity exceeding 100 percent of the velocity in the proximal vessel (in practice, this implies a peak systolic velocity of >200 cm/s); and loss of the reverse-flow component, producing a high-velocity, monophasic waveform with continuous diastolic flow. There may be marked spectral broadening. Kohler et al.[2] compared duplex imaging with arteriography and demonstrated a sensitivity of 82 percent and a specificity of 92 percent in identifying lesions with more than 50 percent reduction in diameter.

The manifestations of severe disease on DCI consist of luminal narrowing exceeding 50 percent, visualization of a high-velocity jet showing white coloration with or without blue coloration due to aliasing, persistence of color during diastole, visual bruit (produced by perivascular tissue vibration), and the presence of post-stenotic turbulence seen as a color mosine. Multiple collateral channels may also be identified. Distal to a significant stenosis, damped monophasic waveforms are seen; these appear on DCI as a glowing red artery compared with the peak systolic flashing of red to white with a blue flash during diastole seen in the normal artery. In a comparison of color Doppler imaging with contrast arteriography in determining stenoses with more than 50 percent reduction in diameter, Cossman et al.[3] found that color Doppler demonstrated a sensitivity of 87 percent and a specificity of 99 percent.

EVALUATION FOR ANGIOPLASTY

Individuals best suited for angioplasty exhibit focal stenoses affecting short arterial segments.[4] Poor candidates for angioplasty are those with long stenotic segments better suited for arterial bypass grafting. Figure 4-6 shows images of a suitable patient for angioplasty. DCI demonstrated a distal superficial femoral artery (SFA) stenosis in a 66-year-old patient with bilateral calf claudication. Proximal to the focal stenosis the waveform is triphasic, indicating absence of significant proximal disease. Dampened waveforms are seen immediately proximal to the stenosis. In the region of Hunter's canal is a tight stenosis producing peak systolic velocities exceeding 300 cm/s with marked diastolic flow. There is loss of the reverse-flow component. Distal to this focal stenosis, the waveforms are dampened and monophasic, suggesting the presence of proximal disease. In view of the short segment involved, this focal stenosis was amenable to balloon dilatation. The results were documented the following day by repeat pulsed Doppler and DCI (Fig. 4-7). The waveforms at and distal to the prior stenosis are dramatically better than those before angioplasty, although some minimal flow disturbance is seen on DCI.

Similar improvements can be seen after atherectomy. A 73-year-old patient with severe left calf claudication was found to have a 15-mm occlusion of the distal left SFA by DCI

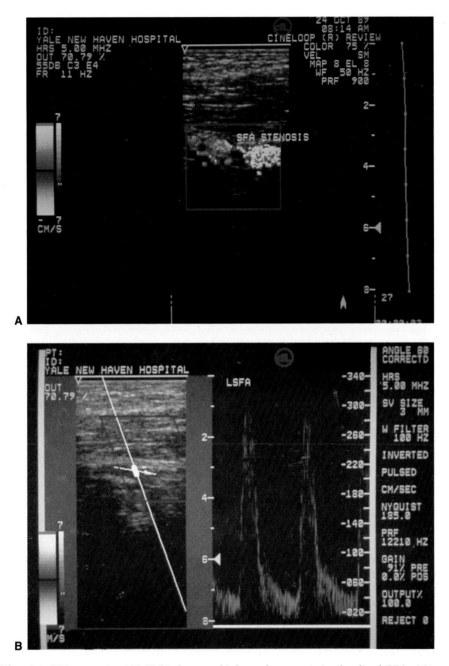

Fig. 4-6 SFA stenosis. **(A)** DCI shows a high-grade stenosis in the distal SFA. Note the poststenotic turbulence seen as a color mosaic. **(B)** Doppler waveforms obtained at the stenosis demonstrate a monophasic waveform with high peak systolic velocities and loss of the reverse-flow component.

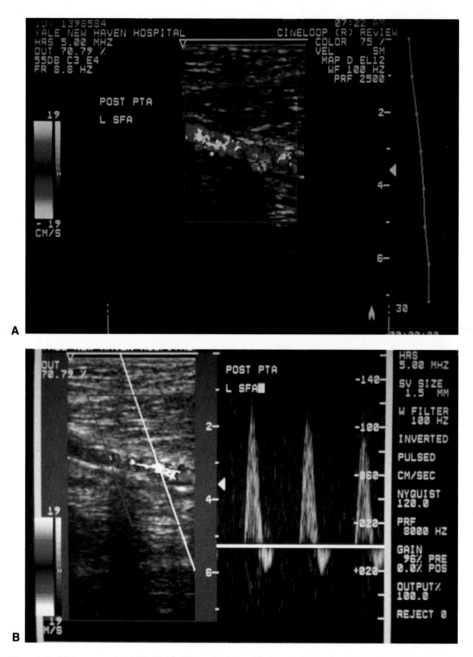

Fig. 4-7 SFA stenosis. **(A)** DCI following angioplasty shows a persistent mosaic pattern compatible with mild turbulence. **(B)** Pulsed-Doppler spectral waveforms demonstrate return of the reverse-flow component in diastole and the peak systolic velocity in the normal range.

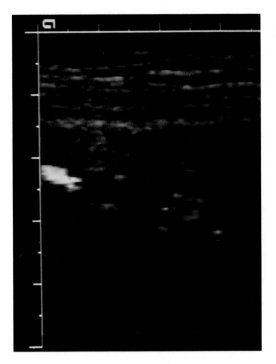

Fig. 4-8 SFA occlusion. DCI image demonstrates a short occlusion of the distal SFA prior to atherectomy.

(Fig. 4-8). Pullback atherectomy was performed. Repeat color Doppler examination demonstrates a patent SFA (Fig. 4-9).

VEIN MAPPING FOR BYPASS GRAFTS

Preoperative mapping of the saphenous veins prior to in situ bypass grafting is helpful in planning and executing bypass procedures.[5,6] The addition of DCI equipment greatly expedites determination of vein size and patency as well as the location of valve cusps. The position of the long saphenous vein can be recorded rapidly, and the presence of branches can be documented. In addition, the valve cusps can clearly be seen by the high-resolution ultrasound imaging now available (Fig. 4-10). Some surgeons argue that because the anatomy of the long saphenous veins is relatively constant, color-flow mapping is unnecessary. However, knowledge of the precise position of the vein allows smaller skin flaps to harvest the vein and

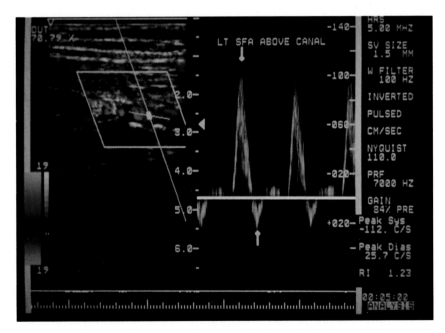

Fig. 4-9 SFA occlusion. The same vessel as shown in Figure 4-8 is shown following pullback atherectomy. Patency is restored, and a normal triphasic waveform is seen.

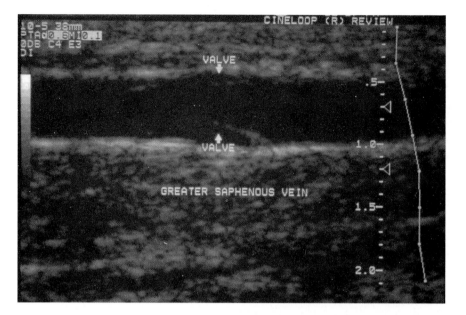

Fig. 4-10 Venous valves. Valve cups are clearly identified on high-resolution images.

decreases the morbidity associated with sloughing of skin flaps.

EVALUATION OF GRAFT PATENCY

Increasing application of vascular surgical techniques has resulted in considerable innovation for revascularization of limbs in which viability is jeopardized by severe vascular disease. Unfortunately, all surgical grafts have a significant incidence of subsequent graft occlusion, and surveillance is required to document patency. Duplex Doppler was found to be more reliable than the ankle/brachial index (ABI) in identifying failing grafts.[7] The combination of an abnormal ABI and duplex scan was associated with increased risk of graft occlusion.[8] Color and duplex Doppler examination should be performed immediately postoperatively to provide a baseline demonstrating normal flow within the graft. Follow-up examinations are then performed at 3-month intervals for the first 2 years and then at 6-month intervals. The rationale for such close surveillance is that grafts do not occlude suddenly, but instead exhibit progressive narrowing and reduction of the flow rate, which lead to eventual occlusion. Thus, timely detection of increasing stenosis in a graft allows appropriate management by angioplasty instead of relentless progression to occlusion. Turbulence is normally seen at proximal anastomoses. A 100 percent increase in velocity is a criterion for significant stenosis. Bandyk et al.[9,10] showed that peak systolic flow velocities below 45 cm/s identified bypass grafts with impending occlusion. In a recent study using color Doppler imaging,[11] a sensitivity of 95 percent and a specificity of 100 percent were achieved in the detection of focal graft stenoses with greater than 50 percent diameter reduction.

For evaluation of graft patency, the entire graft as well as the proximal and distal vessels must be examined by DCI and pulsed Doppler (Fig. 4-11). It is important to compare graft diameters at inflow and outflow sites

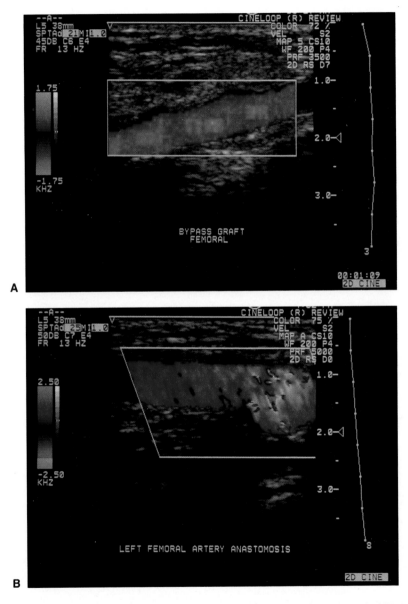

Fig. 4-11 Femoral bypass graft. **(A)** DCI demonstrates patent bypass graft. **(B)** Image of the distal anastomotic site shows a characteristic flow disturbance.

to avoid misclassifying increased velocities as stenoses.[12]

ANEURYSMAL DISEASE

In Western culture, the vast majority of aneurysms are atherosclerotic. Aneurysms affecting flow to the lower limbs include those originating in the aorta, the iliac artery, and the popliteal artery. DCI imaging of aneurysms shows very complex flow patterns with a central jet and often very slow reversed flow around the periphery. In view of this low-flow state, it is not surprising that mural thrombus is common. In this situation, DCI is most helpful. Gray-scale images demonstrate the aneurysmal shell and the intraluminal clot, whereas DCI demonstrates the residual lumen through the aneurysm (Fig. 4-12).

PSEUDOANEURYSMS

Pseudoaneurysms have been found in many different arteries, but they usually occur in the femoral artery as a result of cardiac catheterization. The presenting symptom is a pulsating inguinal mass. The differential diagnosis includes pseudoaneurysm, arteriovenous fistula, and hematoma overlying the femoral artery. DCI examination demonstrates a jet of blood entering the pseudoaneurysm during systole. This jet impinges against the far wall of the pseudoaneurysm and reverses down the side walls to reenter the artery during diastole owing to a change in pressure within the pseudoaneurysm. Thus, a pulsed-Doppler sample volume placed over the communicating neck of the pseudoaneurysm shows typical "to-and-fro" motion (Fig. 4-13).[13]

The surgeon needs to know whether the mass is a pseudoaneurysm or a hematoma. DCI can reliably distinguish a pseudoaneurysm from a hematoma, rendering confirmatory angiography unnecessary. DCI can also determine the position of the neck of the pseudoaneurysm for definitive surgical repair.

A recent report documented successful treatment of pseudoaneurysms by prolonged application of pressure over the communicating neck.[14] Sufficient pressure is exerted by the transducer to obliterate the cavity of the pseudoaneurysm while flow is maintained in the underlying artery. After 10 minutes, the pressure is relieved and the color-flow image

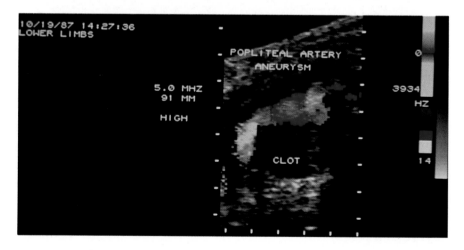

Fig. 4-12 Popliteal artery aneurysm. Note the narrow lumen and marked mural thrombus.

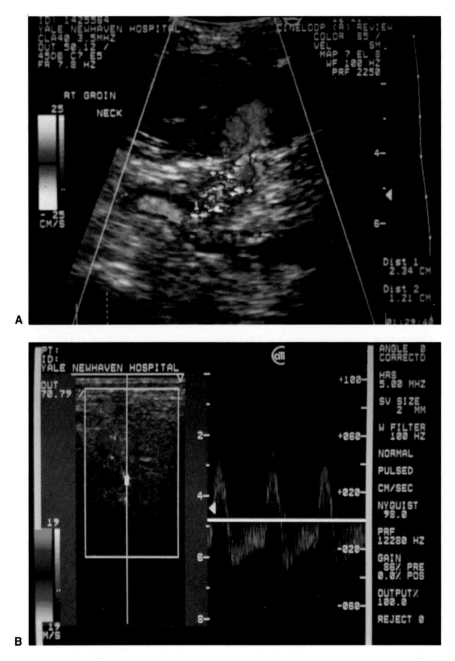

Fig. 4-13 Femoral artery pseudoaneurysm. **(A)** DCI demonstrates the wide neck of the pseudoaneurysm and moderate surrounding hematoma. **(B)** Duplex examination demonstrates typical "to-and-fro" flow pattern.

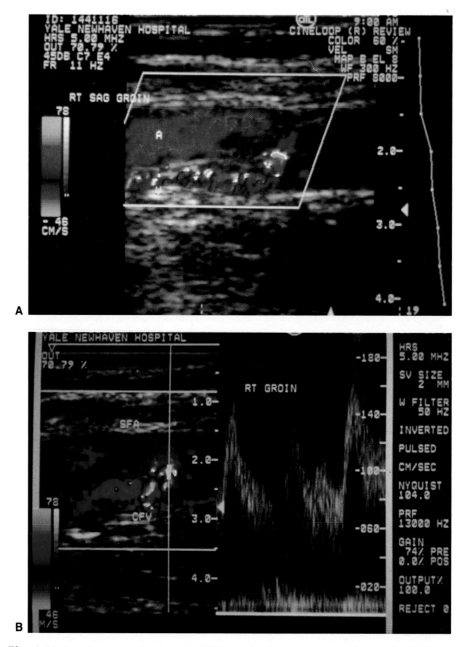

Fig. 4-14 Arteriovenous fistula. **(A)** DCI clearly shows a communication between artery and vein following femoral puncture. Marked turbulence is identified in the draining vein. **(B)** Doppler interrogation of the fistula demonstrates turbulent, continuous low-impedance flow pattern.

checked to see whether there is persistent flow in the pseudoaneurysm. If the pseudoaneurysm persists, the procedure is repeated for three or four subsequent 10-minute periods. This therapy is particularly successful for new pseudoaneurysms before endothelialization has occurred.

The clinical application of color Doppler to pseudoaneurysms is particularly successful. Not only does it preclude repeat angiography in patients who have already suffered iatrogenic injury from arteriography, but also it may preclude the need for surgical repair.

ARTERIOVENOUS FISTULAE

Abnormal communications between arteries and veins may result from congenital vascular malformations, knife wounds, or gunshot wounds. Because of the pressure gradient between the artery and vein, there is continuous forward flow, unlike the flow into a pseudoaneurysm[15] (Fig. 4-14). Persistent arterial flow is best seen during diastole. Turbulence at the site of the fistula results in vibration of the vessel wall and perivascular color-flow artifact. With large fistulae, arterial flow into the venous system produces pulsatile flow in the draining vein, and massive arteriovenous shunting may occur, elevating cardiac output to more than 20 L/min.

PITFALLS

Several pitfalls must be considered to avoid misdiagnosis. Loss of reversal of flow in diastole may be caused by reactive hyperemia, limb warming, or exercise, as well as ischemia. The Doppler examination should be performed at rest. An incorrect Doppler angle can falsely elevate velocities. It also may be difficult to distinguish between a high-grade stenosis and occlusion if flow is very slow. Collateral vessels may be mis-

taken for major arteries. Collaterals may cross over other vessels, producing confusing or unusual waveforms. Finally, it should be remembered that turbulence may be identified following intervention.

Color velocity scale settings must also be set appropriately. A mistaken impression of occlusion can be made if the color velocity scale is set too high. Conversely, focal color changes due to aliasing can be mistaken as stenoses if the color velocity scale is set too low. Although vascular calcification may impair visualization of the vessel walls and duplex examination, lack of focal color changes and increased flow velocities at the distal portion of the visualized vessel suggest the absence of a significant stenosis.

SUMMARY

The impact of DCI on the evaluation of peripheral vascular disease is considerable. In essence, it is noninvasive angiography without the limitations of that modality. However, the pressure gradient can only be inferred, and pull-through pressure gradients are still the most accurate estimation of adequacy of flow. Nonetheless, segmental blood pressures and the peak velocities measured by duplex Doppler provide a noninvasive alternative for estimating pressure gradients. DCI imaging has greatly improved the perception of focal abnormalities and allows rapid appreciation of global hemodynamics. As further technical refinements improve resolution and sensitivity, color Doppler may eventually supplant angiography as the primary imaging modality in peripheral arterial diagnosis, reserving arteriography for interventional procedures.

REFERENCES

1. Jager KA, Phillips DJ, Martin RL, et al: Noninvasive mapping of lower limb arterial lesions. Ultrasound Med Biol 11:515, 1985

2. Kohler TR, Nance DR, Cramer MM, et al: Duplex scanning for diagnosis of aortoiliac and femoropopliteal disease: a prospective study. Circulation 76:1074, 1987

3. Cossman DV, Ellison JE, Wagner WH, et al: Comparison of contrast arteriography to arterial mapping with color-flow duplex imaging in the lower extremities. J Vasc Surg 10:522, 1989

4. Edwards JM, Coldwell DM, Goldman ML, Strandness DE Jr: The role of duplex scanning in the selection of patients for transluminal angioplasty. J Vasc Surg 13:69, 1991

5. Leopold PW, Shandall AA, Corson JD, et al: Initial experience comparing B-mode imaging and venography of the saphenous vein before in situ bypass. Am J Surg 152:206, 1986

6. Fitzgerald KM, Kupinski AM, Kay C, et al: B-mode ultrasound vein mapping. J Vasc Technol 12:62, 1988

7. Mills JL, Harris EJ, Taylor LM Jr, et al: The importance of routine surveillance of distal bypass grafts with duplex scanning: a study of 379 reversed vein grafts. J Vasc Surg 12:379, 1990

8 Green RM, McNamara J, Ouriel K, DeWeese JA: Comparison of infrainguinal graft surveillance techniques. J Vasc Surg 11:207, 1990

9. Bandyk DF, Kaebnick HW, Bergamini TM, et al: Hemodynamics of in-situ saphenous vein arterial bypass. Arch Surg 123:477, 1988

10. Bandyk DF, Seabrook GR, Moldenhauer P, et al: Hemodynamics of vein graft stenoses. J Vasc Surg 8:688, 1988

11. Polak JF, Donaldson MC, Dobkin GR, et al: Early detection of saphenous vein arterial bypass graft stenosis by color-assisted duplex sonography: a prospective study. AJR 154:857, 1990

12. Londrey GL, Hodgson KJ, Spadone DP, et al: Initial experience with color-flow duplex scanning of infrainguinal bypass grafts. J Vasc Surg 12:284, 1990

13. Mitchell DG, Needleman L, Bezzi M, et al: Femoral artery pseudoaneurysm: diagnosis with conventional duplex and color Doppler US. Radiology 165:687, 1987

14. Fellmeth BD, Roberts AC, Bookstein JJ, et al: Postangiographic femoral artery injuries: nonsurgical repair with US-guided compression. Radiology 178:671, 1991

15. Igidbashian VN, Mitchell DG, Middleton WD, et al: Iatrogenic femoral arteriovenous fistula: diagnosis with color Doppler imaging. Radiology 170:749, 1989

5

Evaluation of Peripheral Venous Disease

Christopher R. B. Merritt

Deep venous thrombosis (DVT) is a major medical problem, and undiagnosed DVT is thought to be responsible for the majority of the 600,000 cases of pulmonary embolism that are estimated to occur in the United States each year.[1,2] On the basis of clinical findings alone, the diagnosis of DVT is considered to be unreliable and the true incidence of DVT is believed to be significantly greater than that detected clinically.[3-6] The importance of a correct diagnosis of DVT is great—failure to diagnose thrombosis may lead to fatal pulmonary embolism, whereas a false-positive diagnosis may expose the patient to the risk of unnecessary anticoagulation. In the past, the diagnostic evaluation of the venous system for occlusive and thromboembolic disease relied on invasive angiographic methods. Today, however, noninvasive approaches to the evaluation of the nervous system by using ultrasonography have assumed a primary diagnostic role. Doppler color imaging (DCI) is a particularly important addition to the methods for

rapid and effective identification of DVT. The proven value of ultrasound has, in turn, diminished reliance on other noninvasive methods including impedance plethysmography, radionuclide venography, and radionuclide fibrinogen scanning. With many studies indicating that the sensitivity and specificity of ultrasound for the detection of DVT are in the range of 90 to 100 percent compared with venography, ultrasound is now well established as the primary noninvasive method for venous evaluation in patients suspected of having DVT.

The success of ultrasound in general and DCI in particular for the diagnosis of venous thrombosis has raised serious questions about the value of venography as the gold standard for diagnosis of lower extremity DVT. Today the use of ultrasound for initial evaluation of patients suspected of having DVT is being increasingly recommended, and venography is reserved for situations that require additional confirmation. It is now proper to consider ultrasound the procedure of choice in the initial assessment of patients suspected of having DVT and venous reflux.

Several ultrasonographic approaches to diagnosis of DVT have been described as effective, including high-resolution ultrasound imaging, duplex Doppler ultrasonography, and DCI.[7-9] These studies have based the diagnosis of DVT on morphologic and dynamic features of the vessels being evaluated. DCI permits visual identification of blood flow, and recent studies confirm an important role for this form of ultrasound in the evaluation of venous disease.[10-13]

PATHOPHYSIOLOGY OF DEEP VENOUS THROMBOSIS

DVT develops under conditions of endothelial damage, flow stasis, and a hypercoagulable state (Virchow's triad). Platelets and fibrin accumulate in the apex of the valve recess (Fig. 5-1); this is followed by the development of inflammation and the formation of thrombus, which becomes vascularized or organized. Thrombus then extends into the vein lumen, producing turbulence. Further growth of the thrombus may lead to obstruction of the vein. With stasis due to obstruction there is rapid retrograde and antegrade propagation of thrombus. During recanalization of the thrombus, contraction of the thrombus renders the valves incompetent, leading to reflux.

Conditions associated with increased risk for DVT are

Congestive heart failure
Varicosities of the lower extremities
Trauma, severe burns
Postpartum
Widespread malignancy

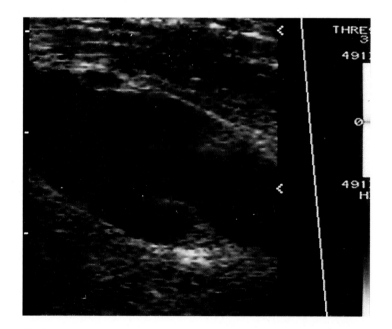

Fig. 5-1 Early deep venous thrombosis. Small slightly echogenic thrombi are present in the apex of the valve recess of the SFV. The thrombus prevents complete opening of the valve, producing turbulent flow and stasis that contribute to propagation of the thrombus.

The most common site for involvement is in the deep calf veins. These are estimated to be involved in 95 percent of patients. Next are the femoral veins (60 percent), followed by the popliteal and iliac veins. The risk of embolus, the major life-threatening complication of DVT, is associated with the degree of venous obstruction and the size of the emboli. Large emboli from the femoral and iliac veins are more likely to be lethal. It is also thought that embolization from a partially occluded vein is more likely than from one that is totally occluded. The risk of symptomatic pulmonary emboli from DVT isolated to the calf veins is slight. Although embolism is the major complication of DVT, the development of valvular incompetence is another significant complication that may result from DVT. Valvular incompetence may lead to reverse flow through perforating veins, collateral circulation through superficial veins, and increased pressure in superficial veins, leading to varicosities and cutaneous ulceration. Early diagnosis and treatment are therefore critical in preventing these serious complications of DVT.

The clinical manifestations of DVT are nonspecific and include edema, pain, and tenderness. Edema is most often associated with occlusive thrombi of the major draining veins of the extremity, usually in the upper leg. Edema may not be present when the thrombosis is restricted to isolated veins in the lower leg owing to the presence of collateral pathways. Extremity pain and tenderness may result from vein distension due to the thrombus, swelling due to edema, or inflammatory changes in the vessel. The clinical diagnosis of DVT is complicated because extensive DVT may be present without symptoms if there is no edema or inflammation. The clinical signs are nonspecific and are therefore unreliable; the diagnostic sensitivity of an experience examiner has been estimated to be only about 50 percent.[14] Thus a significant problem arises since patients with minimal symptoms may harbor extensive DVT while 50 to 70 percent of patients with signs and symptoms suggesting DVT have normal veins. Also, as a result of the prevalence of minimal symptoms, it is likely that the true incidence of DVT is significantly greater than clinically suspected. Failure to identify a major DVT may lead to fatal pulmonary embolism or be followed by the long-term problems associated with chronic venous insufficiency, thus heightening this clinical dilemma. Therefore, early and accurate diagnosis is of great importance in this problem.

ANATOMY

The veins of the lower extremity include superficial and deep vessels, as well as communicating veins in the calf (Fig. 5-2). The deep veins include the common, superficial, and deep femoral veins; the popliteal vein; and the anterior tibial, peroneal, and posterior tibial veins of the calf. The superficial veins include the greater and lesser saphenous veins. The superficial and deep venous systems are connected by communicating veins, most numerous between the distal greater saphenous vein and the posterior tibial vein in the calf. The greatest risk of pulmonary embolism is from thrombosis arising in the deep venous system. The vessels most commonly implicated in lower extremity venous thrombosis are the common femoral, superficial femoral, popliteal, and major calf veins in the deep venous system and the greater saphenous vein in the superficial system. The deep veins follow the course of the femoral artery and its branches. The anatomic relationship of the artery to the accompanying vein changes as the vessels pass distally. The femoral artery and vein enter the upper thigh from beneath the inguinal ligament. In this location the femoral vein lies medial to the artery. Deep and superficial branches of the femoral vein follow the corresponding major branches of the femoral artery. Distal to the bifurcation of the femoral vein the superficial

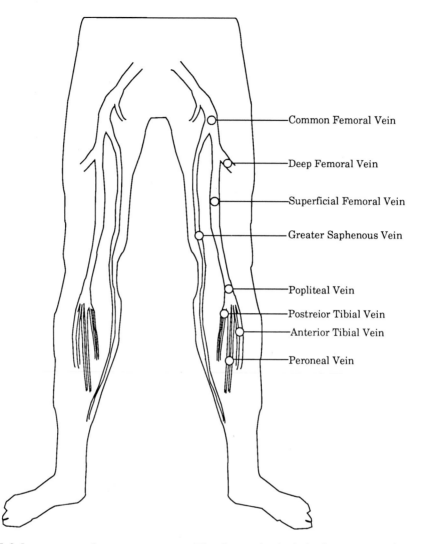

Fig. 5-2 Lower extremity venous system. The deep veins include the common femoral, superficial femoral, and deep femoral veins; the popliteal vein; and the paired anterior tibial, peroneal, and posterior tibial veins of the calf. The superficial veins include the greater and lesser saphenous (not shown) veins. The superficial and deep venous systems are connected by communicating veins, most numerous between the distal greater saphenous vein and the posterior tibial vein in the calf.

femoral vein (SFV) passes posterior (deep) to the femoral artery (Fig. 5-3A). Near the junction of the SFV and the deep femoral vein both veins may be imaged, but more distally only the superficial femoral vein is seen (Fig. 5-3B). As the superficial femoral artery and SFV approach the knee, both vessels deviate medially and deeply into the adductor canal, passing between the distal portion of the adductor magnus and the vastus medialis. In this location the SFV is quite deep, and in many patients this makes examination by imaging and compression difficult or impossible. Indirect testing aids in confirming

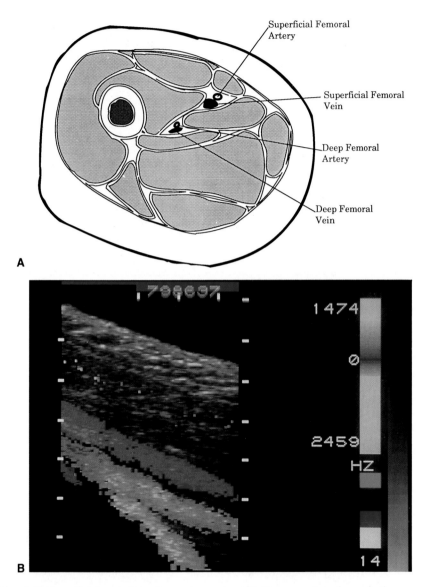

Fig. 5-3 Superficial and deep femoral vessels. **(A)** Cross section through the upper thigh just distal to the bifurcation of the common femoral artery shows the relationships of the superficial and deep femoral veins to their respective arteries. **(B)** Longitudinal DCI in the upper thigh shows the common, superficial, and deep femoral veins (blue). At this location the veins lie deep or slightly medial to the arteries. Near the junction of the superficial and deep femoral veins, both veins may be imaged, but more distally only the SFV is seen.

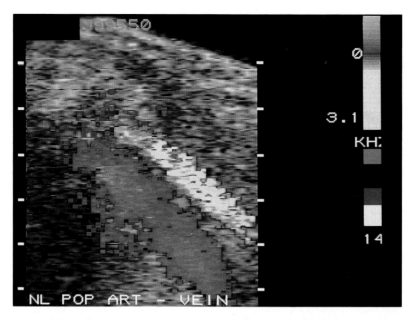

Fig. 5-4 Normal popliteal vein and artery. Scan from the posterior aspect of the popliteal fossa shows the popliteal vein (blue) as it lies slightly medial and posterior (superficial) to the popliteal artery (red).

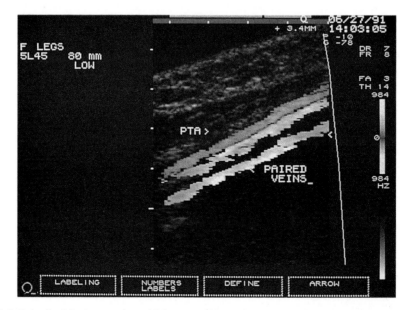

Fig. 5-5 Paired calf veins. In the calf the arterial branches are usually accompanied by paired veins. Here the posterior tibial artery and its two accompanying veins are shown. Although difficult to demonstrate by conventional imaging, these small vessels may be demonstrated easily by DCI.

the patency of this segment of the SFV. The popliteal vein lies slightly medial and posterior (superficial) to the popliteal artery (Fig. 5-4). Distal to the knee, the popliteal artery gives off an anterior tibial branch and divides into the peroneal and posterior tibial arteries. Branches of the popliteal veins accompany these arteries, usually in pairs, with two venous branches accompanying each of the arterial branches into the calf (Fig. 5-5). The normal relationships of arteries and veins are important because the artery is the main landmark used to locate the accompanying vein. Failure to visualize a vein in its expected location is an important clue to venous thrombosis.

In addition to the deep venous system, the greater and lesser saphenous veins should also be evaluated. The lesser saphenous vein runs along the lateral aspect of the calf and drains into the popliteal vein. The greater saphenous vein lies along the medial aspect of the calf and thigh, just beneath the subcutaneous tissues, and empties into the femoral vein just proximal to the junction of the SFV and deep femoral vein to form the common femoral vein. The superficial femoral, popliteal, and calf veins contain valves along their course. Valves are less common in more proximal locations. Communicating veins connect the superficial and deep veins in the calf and are provided with valves to prevent flow from the deep to the superficial systems.

EXAMINATION TECHNIQUE

Complete ultrasound assessment of the venous system of the lower extremity should include examination of all segments of the deep veins.[15] Evaluation of the greater saphenous vein and the proximal portion of the deep femoral vein is also necessary because thrombus in the proximal portions of these vessels is a potential source of emboli. Although there is general agreement about the sensitivity and specificity of ultrasound in the detection of thrombus in the larger vessels

above the calf, the ability of ultrasound to detect thrombosis in the calf veins is only partially defined. The clinical importance of thrombus isolated to small calf veins is unclear, although it has been suggested that 20 percent of clots in the calf veins will extend into the larger veins and result in embolism. Our approach using DCI is to routinely image the major calf veins (posterior tibial, peroneal, and anterior tibial) as well as the larger vessels.

The examination is usually begun with the patient supine with the hip slightly abducted and externally rotated to allow access to the inner aspect of the thigh. The common and superficial femoral veins and greater saphenous veins are examined with the patient supine. For evaluation of the popliteal and calf veins, the patient is placed in the lateral decubitis or prone position. Elevation of the head of the bed to 10 or 15 degrees may aid in the examination by distending the veins of interest. Attempts to visualize the SFV within the adductor canal should be made, but this may not always be possible, particularly in large or obese patients. Depending on patient size and equipment, imaging is usually performed with 5.0- or 7.5-MHz transducers. In obese patients or those with severe swelling of the extremity, adequate penetration of deeper vein segments may require 3.0-MHz imaging frequencies. Rather than use the same frequency throughout the examination, we prefer to change transducers, using higher-frequency transducers to evaluate more superficial veins, attempting to visualize valve areas for subtle disturbances, and using lower frequencies as necessary to image areas not adequately shown with higher frequencies.

There is considerable variation in the normal flow velocity of blood in lower extremity veins, and velocities ranging from greater than 20 cm/s to less than 1 cm/s may be encountered. Because of the relatively slow flow encountered in many patients, it is extremely important that the instrument se-

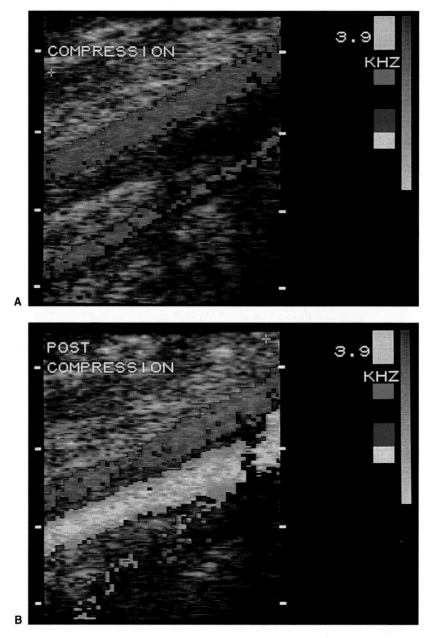

Fig. 5-6 Enhancement maneuvers—compression. **(A)** Images of the SFV show complete collapse with compression by the transducer. The compressed SFV lies between the superficial femoral artery and deep femoral artery (both shown in red). **(B)** Release of compression is accompanied by flow that completely fills the vessel lumen, confirming absence of thrombosis. Augmented flow is also noted after gentle compression of the soft tissues of the extremity distal to the examination site. (*Figure continues.*)

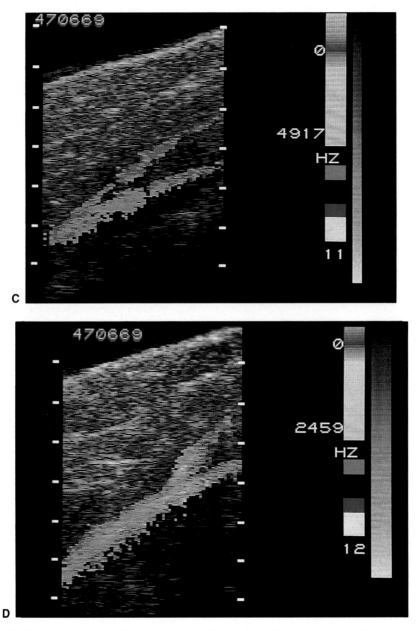

Fig. 5-6 (*Continued*). **(C)** Resting flow at the saphenofemoral junction. **(D)** Augmented flow at this junction is shown when the distal extremity is compressed. Observation of augmented flow after compression maneuvers is a simple and rapid means of confirming vein patency.

lected for the examination have good sensitivity for the detection of slow flow. Instrument settings should be carefully adjusted as recommended by the manufacturer to provide optimal detection of normal slow venous flow. As in other Doppler vascular studies, to maintain sensitivity it is important to use a Doppler angle of less than 60 degrees between the ultrasound beam and the direction of flow within the vessel. This is particularly important when evaluating slow venous flow because a large Doppler angle will result in marked reduction of the detected Doppler frequency shift and may suggest absence of flow altogether. The proper selection of instrument settings, use of a proper Doppler angle, and application of flow augmentation maneuvers described below will permit visualization of most if not all normal vessels. Finally, scanning should be performed with extremely light pressure to avoid inadvertent compression of the vein. To identify vessels quickly, imaging in the transverse plane followed by longitudinal imaging is used to map the vessel course.

The examination is begun in a transverse imaging plane at or slightly above the inguinal ligament with identification of the distal external iliac vein and artery. To detect slow venous flow, the transducer is angled cephalad to produce a suitable angle between the flow direction and the ultrasound beam. Applying minimal pressure, the transducer is moved down the medial aspect of the thigh, following the course of the superficial femoral artery and SFV. This quick initial examination is sufficient to provide evidence of gross pathologic charges in the femoral vein and to show the position of the vessels for more detailed examination in longitudinal imaging planes. Patency of the common femoral vein and SFV is established by direct inspection. In thin patients a considerable segment of the external iliac vein is also visible. Scanning through a distended urinary bladder may permit examination of the iliac veins. The patency of nonvisualized portions of the iliac veins may be inferred by observing the effects of respiration and Valsalva maneuver on flow dynamics in the femoral vein. In patients unable to perform the Valsalva maneuver, manual compression of the abdomen may be helpful. With Valsalva or firm compression of the abdomen, flow in the femoral vein ceases, and when compression or Valsalva is released, augmented flow results. These normal dynamics are absent or reduced in the presence of iliac vein occlusion. It is important to note that the diagnosis of mild degrees of partial thrombosis of the iliac vein probably cannot be made from these indirect tests. Lower extremity veins are examined during resting flow and during a variety of flow augmentation maneuvers. These maneuvers include direct venous compression and relaxation by using the transducer as a compression device, mild compression of the extremity distal to the transducer to enhance venous flow rates, and respiratory maneuvers including deep inspirations and expirations, Valsalva maneuvers, and abdominal compression (Figs. 5-6 and 5-7). The examination technique for visualizing the calf veins involves identifying the anterior tibial, posterior tibial, and peroneal arteries in transverse planes at the level of the mid calf. Then, with the patient supine, an anterolateral approach between the tibia and fibula allows imaging of the anterior tibial and peroneal vessels (Fig. 5-8). A posteromedial approach is used to visualize the posterior tibial and peroneal vessels. Veins accompanying the arteries are identified with compression augmentation by gently squeezing the distal calf or foot. Using the techniques described above, an experienced examiner can perform a thorough DCI examination of the lower extremity venous system in 5 to 10 minutes for each leg.

DIAGNOSTIC CRITERIA FOR DEEP VENOUS THROMBOSIS

Currently there are three methods for using ultrasound in the identification of DVT. These are imaging alone, duplex

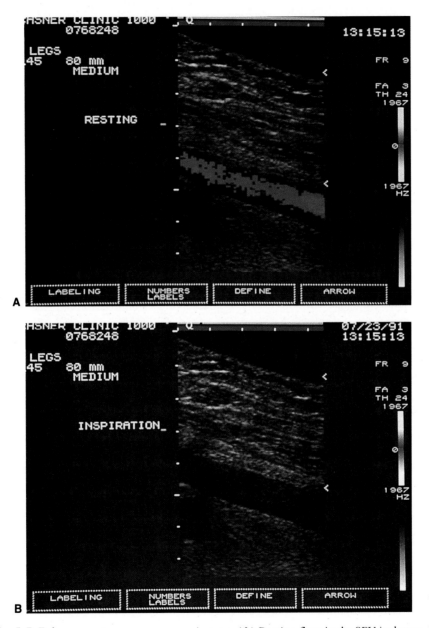

Fig. 5-7 Enhancement maneuvers—respiratory. **(A)** Resting flow in the SFV is shown. Low velocity flow near the vein wall results in incomplete filling of the vessel lumen with color. **(B)** During inspiration there is cessation of flow in the SFV. (*Figure continues.*)

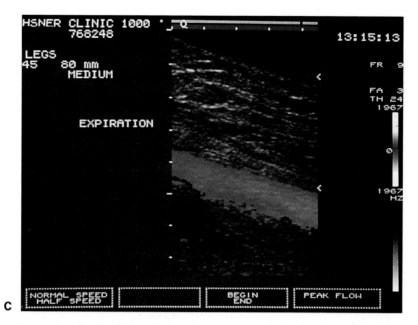

Fig. 5-7 (*Continued*). **(C)** With expiration there is increased flow within the SFV, aiding in confirmation of patency.

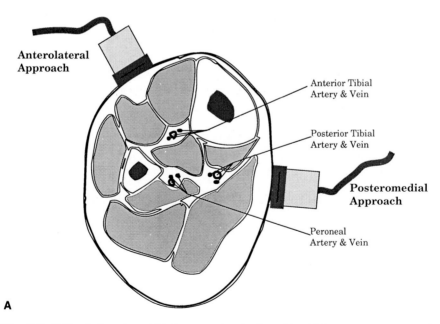

Fig. 5-8 Calf vein imaging. **(A)** Cross section in the mid-calf demonstrates approaches for imaging the calf veins. (*Figure continues.*)

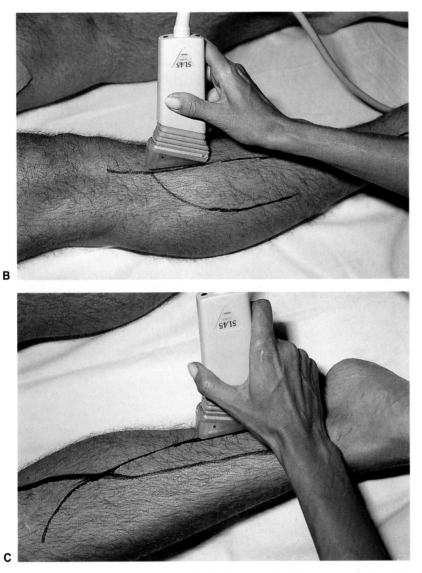

Fig. 5-8 (*Continued*). **(B)** The anterior tibial and peroneal veins are seen by imaging from an anterolateral approach. **(C)** The posterior tibial and peroneal veins are imaged by using a posteromedial approach.

Doppler, and DCI. DCI employs elements of both imaging and duplex ultrasound, and diagnostic criteria overlap with those used for imaging and duplex examination.

Imaging Criteria

VISUALIZATION OF THROMBUS

The earliest manifestation of DVT detectable by ultrasound is the finding of small areas of thrombus in the valve recess (Fig. 5-1). This is a subtle finding, demonstrable only with high-resolution imaging equipment. DCI may show flow disturbances associated with these early changes (Fig. 5-9). As the thrombus enlarges and propagates within the vein, flow disturbances and loss of vein compressibility are present. A limitation of the criterion of thrombus visualization is, of course,

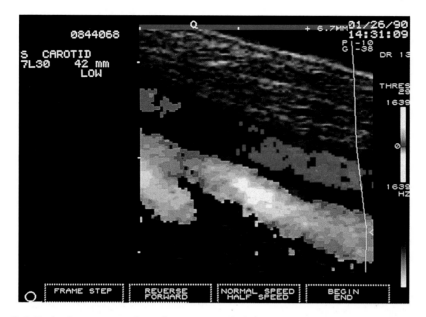

Fig. 5-9 Early deep venous thrombosis. A small thrombus in the valve recess is seen in a patient with early DVT. DCI shows a flow void due to thrombus preventing complete opening of the valve.

that all thrombi are not sufficiently echogenic to be readily identified by imaging alone. Also, artifact, especially in small vessels, may give rise to intraluminal echoes that suggest the presence of thrombus when none is present. With DCI, imaging information is coupled with information related to flow, overcoming this problem. The imaging of flow provides contrast within the vessel lumen and enhances the visibility of hypoechoic thrombi, which appears as areas of flow void within the vessel (Fig. 5-10). Increased velocity in areas of narrowing produced by partially occluding thrombi is also seen (Fig. 5-11).

VEIN COMPRESSIBILITY

Normal veins have thin walls and are easily compressed. The lack of compressibility is an important imaging criterion for the presence of intraluminal thrombus. Venous compression should be applied while a trans-verse image of the vein is obtained to prevent the possibility of the transducer slipping off of the vein (Figs. 5-12 and 5-13). The ability to compress the vein completely is generally regarded as a reliable indicator of the absence of thrombus. Since partial compressibility of a vein containing thrombus is possible, the importance of demonstrating complete compressibility is emphasized. Compressibility of the veins in the adductor canal and the common and external iliac veins is difficult or impossible, limiting the imaging assessment of these vessels. An increasingly recognized limitation of the criterion of vein compressibility is the lack of complete compressibility of veins in patients with old DVT. Recanalized veins in patients without acute DVT may have compression characteristics suggesting acute thrombus. DCI is extremely helpful in identification of recanalization of old thrombus and may avoid some of the false-positive diagnoses made with compression imaging.

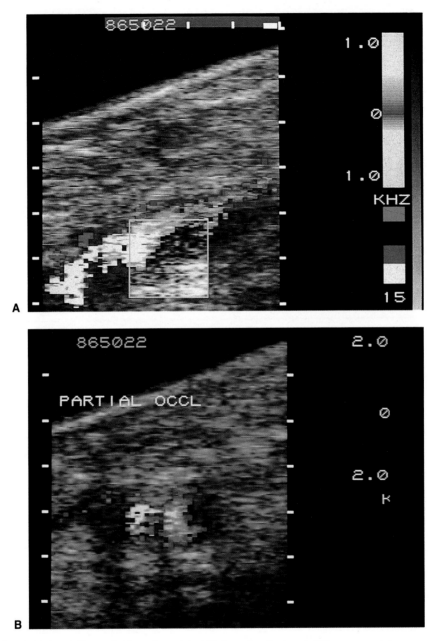

Fig. 5-10 Partially occluding thrombi. **(A)** Longitudinal and **(B)** transverse images of the SFV. Thrombus narrows the lumen of the SFV but does not produce complete occlusion. DCI provides contrast between the vessel wall, thrombus, and lumen and enhances the visibility of hypoechoic thrombi, which appear as areas of flow void within the vessel.

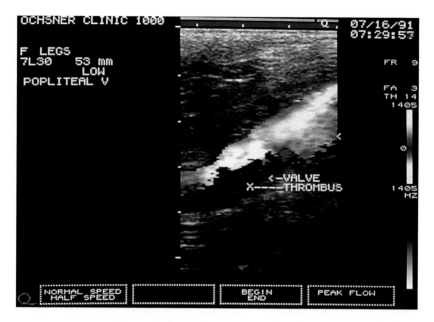

Fig. 5-11 Partially occluding thrombus. In addition to showing the flow void produced by the thrombus, increased velocity is present in areas of narrowing produced by the thrombus.

VEIN SIZE

The presence of thrombus typically enlarges the vein diameter, making the vein appear significantly larger than its accompanying artery. If the thrombus distending the vein is echogenic, DCI is not needed for diagnosis. When the clot is hypoechoic, the use of DCI is helpful in conforming the absence of flow and defining the degree of occlusion.

RESPIRATORY CHANGES

Larger veins increase noticeably in diameter with deep inspiration or with the Valsalva maneuver and diminish in diameter with expiration as abdominal pressure is reduced and flow resumes. Observation of normal respiratory dynamics therefore aids in confirming venous patency. When DCI is performed, direct observation of venous flow and changes in vein diameter is possible. Absence of normal response may indicate occlusion of vessels proximal to the site being examined.

Flow Criteria

SPONTANEOUS FLOW

In large veins spontaneous flow is present at rest. The velocity of blood flow in veins varies considerably among individuals and may be quite low. For this reason, the sensitivity of the Doppler instrument used and the setting of the high-pass filter are of particular importance in ensuring the display of normal slow flow (Fig. 5-14). Usually the high-pass filter of the instrument used will have to be set to the lowest level possible to ensure that low flow velocities are not rejected by the scanner.

PHASIC FLOW AND RESPIRATORY DYNAMICS

Ultrasound methods are unique in their ability to permit the demonstration of normal physiologic changes in flow as indications of venous patency.[8] As noted above, assessment of changes in vein diameter with the Valsalva maneuver and detection of normal

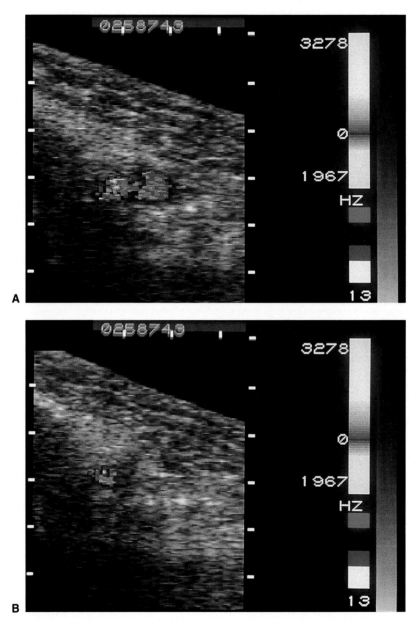

Fig. 5-12 Normal compression. Transverse images of the SFV and superficial femoral artery **(A)** before and **(B)** after compression with the transducer show complete collapse of the vein with pressure. Flow in the superficial femoral artery continues. Venous compression should be applied while a transverse image of the vein is obtained to prevent the possibility of the transducer slipping off of the vein.

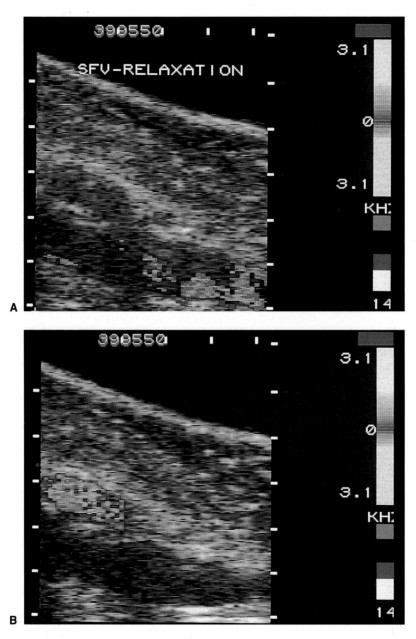

Fig. 5-13 Abnormal compression. **(A)** DCI with augmentation reveals abrupt termination of flow in the SFV. **(B)** With direct compression using the transducer the vein fails to collapse, confirming presence of an occluding thrombus.

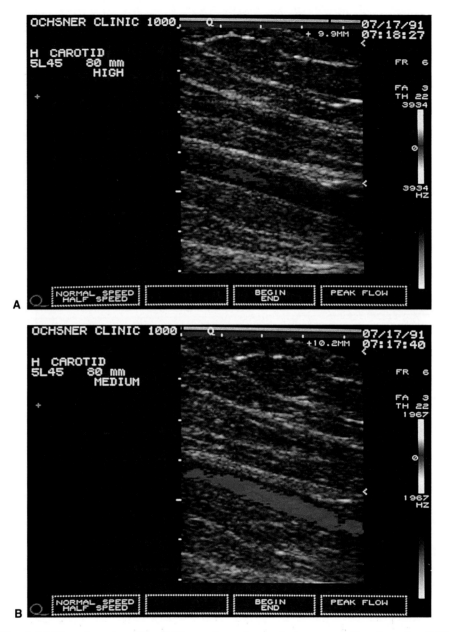

Fig. 5-14 Flow detection. The ability to detect low-velocity venous flow by using DCI is determined by instrument settings. **(A)** The instrument is set to display only high-velocity flow, and flow in the SFV vein is not imaged. **(B)** A medium-sensitivity setting is used, permitting identification of some flow in the vein. (*Figure continues.*)

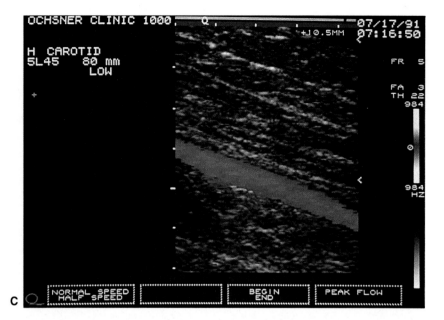

Fig. 5-14 (*Continued*). **(C)** Maximum sensitivity for slow flow detection is used. This allows optimal display of slow venous flow and permits confirmation of flow that might be undetected at higher settings.

venous pulsation are helpful in determining the patency of major veins proximal to the site of evaluation. Although veins are generally thought of as having relatively constant flow, there is a normal variation in flow velocity that is related to changes in pressures due to respiration. This phasic pattern is diminished or lost as blood passes through recanalized or partially occluded segments and is thus of diagnostic value. Deep inspiration or Valsalva procedure normally results in an abrupt cessation of venous flow in larger veins. This response is shown well with DCI and is helpful in confirming the patency of the veins proximal to the point of Doppler measurement, but it may not differentiate nonocclusive thrombosis. Pulsed-Doppler sampling is helpful in confirming the dynamics of flow patterns imaged by DCI, providing more resolution of subtle temporal variations in flow than the image alone (Fig. 5-15).

FLOW AUGMENTATION

Compression of the extremity distal to the point of Doppler measurement will normally result in an immediate augmentation of flow velocity and is another important method for confirming the patency of the vein between the point of observation and the site of compression. As with the Valsalva maneuver, flow augmentation may be seen not only in normal veins but also in those with partial occlusion or recanalization.

With DCI, the evaluation of flow is facilitated by global Doppler sampling. This is particularly valuable in the calf, where normal veins may not be visible by gray-scale imaging alone. DCI permits rapid identification of these veins, and the meticulous sampling and long examination times necessary for a complete duplex examination are largely eliminated when using DCI. Eccen-

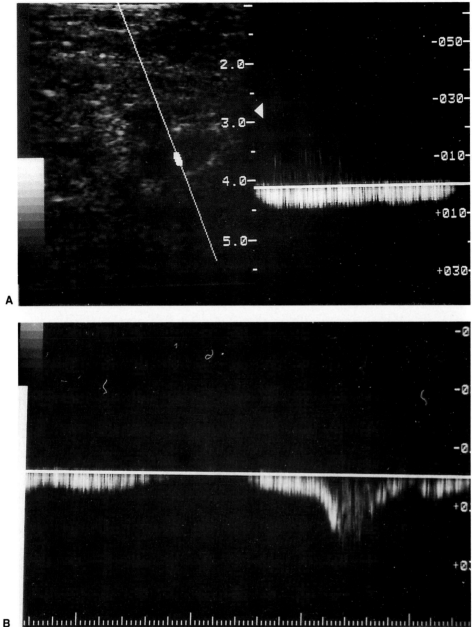

Fig. 5-15 Phasic venous flow. **(A)** Pulsed Doppler spectrum of the SFV shows subtle phasic variations of venous flow related to respiration. **(B)** Flow stops completely during inspiration and resumes with increased velocity in expiration. Pulsed Doppler sampling is helpful in confirming the dynamics of flow patterns imaged by DCI and provides more resolution of subtle temporal variations in flow than does the image alone.

tric thrombus and partially canalized thrombus, difficult to assess by gray-scale imaging and duplex Doppler, can be shown.

EFFICACY OF DOPPLER COLOR IMAGING

A number of studies documenting the efficacy of DCI in venous evaluation of the lower extremities have been published in recent years.[10–13,16] Table 5-1 summarizes the findings in these studies. In 1988, Merritt et al.[10] reported a prospective study of 60 patients referred for evaluation of suspected DVT over a 5-month interval. Fifty-six of these patients also were examined by impedance plethysmography, nine by radionuclide venography, and six by contrast venography by conventional techniques. Lower extremity veins were examined during resting flow and during a variety of flow augmentation maneuvers as described above. In most patients, the iliac veins were also evaluated by scanning along the lateral pelvic wall through the urine-filled bladder. The diagnostic criteria used for the identification of DVT by DCI included direct visualization of thrombus within the vein, loss of flow signal and flow augmentation, and demonstration of collateral vessels accompanying these findings. Additional findings associated with DVT included dilatation of the thrombosed

segment of the vein and loss of normal vein compressibility. On the basis of a combination of clinical findings and venography, DCI, plethysmography, or radionuclide imaging, 19 of the 60 patients evaluated were considered to have sufficient evidence of DVT to warrant treatment with anticoagulation, although only 5 patients had contrast venographic confirmation of abnormality. All 19 patients treated for DVT had positive DCI studies. Of the 19 cases in which DVT was identified, 78.9 percent involved the SFV, 63.2 percent involved the popliteal vein, and 26.3 percent extended into the common femoral vein. No thrombus was found in the iliac veins in this series. On the basis of the clinical decision to treat patients, the sensitivity and specificity of DCI in this study were 100 and 97.6 percent, respectively. There was one false-positive result with DCI, with 19 true positives and 40 true negatives. DCI permitted accurate identification of the location of occluding and nonoccluding thrombi. Of six patients evaluated by venography, both DCI and venography were positive in five and both were negative in the sixth. Because clinicians were aware of the results of the DCI examination, there was considerable reluctance to perform venography in patients with obvious DVT identified by DCI, resulting in lack of venographic correlation for a larger number of patients. More recent studies with larger

Table 5-1 Sensitivity and Specificity of DCI in the Diagnosis of DVT

Source	No. of Patients	Sensitivity (%)	Specificity (%)	Veins Studied
Merritt et al.,[10] 1988	60	96	94	Iliac & femoropopliteal
Foley et al.,[11] 1989	47	100	100	Femoropopliteal
Rose et al.,[17] 1990	75	96	100	Iliac & femoropopliteal
Rose et al.,[17] 1990	75	92	100	Femoropopliteal only
Rose et al.,[17] 1990	75	73	86	Calf only
Rose et al.,[17] 1990	45	95	100	Calf only[a]
Fürst et al.,[16] 1990	102	95	99	Femoropopliteal
Baxter et al.,[12] 1990	40	93	100	Femoropopliteal & calf

[a] Only results of technically adequate studies are included (40 percent of calf studies were considered inadequate).

numbers of venographic studies show similar results.

Foley et al.[11] have reported the results of DCI in a study of 475 patients with suspected lower extremity venous thrombosis. Occlusive and nonocclusive thrombi of the femoral and popliteal veins were detected in 200 (42 percent) of patients. Conventional venography was performed for correlation in 47 patients, confirming 10 cases of femoral popliteal thrombosis, 2 of femoral vein thrombosis, and 7 of isolated popliteal vein thrombosis. DCI and venographic findings agreed in all 12 positive and 35 negative cases involving the femoral veins (100 percent sensitivity and specificity). DCI correctly identified 5 of the 7 isolated popliteal thromboses and all 10 of the femoral popliteal lesions. In discussing their findings, these investigators commented on the value of DCI in demonstrating recanalized segments not identifiable by compression B-mode imaging. In addition, the benefits of DCI in permitting assessment of resting flow without augmentation or reliance on vein compressibility were noted.

Fürst et al.[16] have prospectively compared DCI and venography by performing a total of 102 examinations. In the diagnosis or exclusion of femoropopliteal thrombosis, DCI achieved a sensitivity of 95 percent and a specificity of 99 percent. Baxter et al.[12] have also reported a prospective double-blind study comparing DCI and venography in a group of 40 patients in whom venography was abnormal in 14. There was one false-negative color Doppler scan that missed a calf and lower popliteal thrombosis. These authors reported successful detection of two cases of isolated calf vein thrombosis with DCI. Overall, the sensitivity and specificity for detection of lower limb venous thrombosis, including calf vein assessment, were 93 and 100 percent, respectively.

In 1990, Rose et al.[17] reported on DCI examinations in 75 lower limbs of 69 consecutive patients referred for venographic evaluation of clinically suspected lower extremity DVT. In this study, they attempted to define the performance of DCI in the identification of thrombosis of specific segments of the lower extremity venous system. The DCI study was obtained within 24 hours of the contrast venogram, and studies were interpreted blindly. With contrast venography as the standard for diagnosis of DVT, the overall accuracy of DCI regardless of thrombus size and location or examination quality was 84 percent (sensitivity, 79 percent; specificity, 88 percent). The accuracy of DCI was 99 percent for detection of DVT located above the knee (sensitivity, 96 percent; specificity, 100 percent) and 81 percent for detection of thrombus below the knee (sensitivity, 73 percent; specificity, 86 percent). Approximately 40 percent of examinations of the calf veins were judged to be technically inadequate owing to failure to visualize all portions of the tibioperoneal trunk and posterior tibial and peroneal veins. If only technically adequate examinations of the calf veins were scored, the accuracy of DCI was 98 percent (sensitivity, 95 percent; specificity, 100 percent). In this study, DCI missed three of four small nonocclusive thrombi, a finding of some concern. The authors of this report concluded that the relatively poor overall performance of DCI in detecting calf vein thrombosis was influenced by a 40 percent incidence of technically limited calf examinations, usually related to poor sound penetration arising from profound calf swelling or obesity. When technically adequate examinations of the calf veins were achieved, the diagnostic accuracy of DCI was deemed to be superior to that of other noninvasive methods.

Although there is not general agreement on the necessity of anticoagulation for patients with DVT isolated to calf veins, it is agreed that the identification of calf vein thrombosis is important so that, if treatment is not instituted, follow-up can be performed to ensure that clots do not propagate into the popliteal and femoral veins, when treatment is clearly indicated. The ability of DCI to image normal calf veins and detect isolated calf vein thrombosis is therefore of considerable importance. In addition to the studies discussed above, the efficacy of DCI in identifying normal calf veins has been reported by van Bemmelen et al.[18] and by Polak et al.[13] van Bemmelen et al. were able to visualize all paired veins from the level of the ankle to the popliteal fossa in 30 normal subjects, whereas Polak et al.[13] were able to visualize 98 to 100 percent of posterior tibial veins, 96 to 100 percent of peroneal veins, and 65 percent of anterior tibial veins, leading to the conclusion that DCI can demonstrate patency of posterior tibial and peroneal veins in most patients without DVT and aid in detection of thrombosis below the knee. Visualization of the anterior tibial veins was not correlated with thrombosis.

Although many cases of thrombosis in the common femoral popliteal and proximal portions of the SFV and greater saphenous veins are readily apparent by imaging alone, the addition of flow information by using DCI results in more confident diagnosis when imaging findings are inconclusive. In addition, smaller veins are assessed more accurately by DCI than by imaging alone. The differentiation of acute and chronic veno-occlusive disease by DCI has not been investigated extensively. The sonographic signs of acute and chronic occlusions may overlap somewhat, and with imaging and compression, recanalized veins may be difficult to distinguish from veins containing acute thrombus. Our experience with DCI suggests that recanalization of old thrombus may be recognized by the demonstration of flow channels within the thrombus and may thus be differentiated from acute thrombus. This differentiation is important and may help prevent unnecessary anticoagulation in patients without acute disease.

VENOUS REFLUX

Venous valvular incompetence is an important complication of DVT, resulting from destruction of valves, causing venous stasis, and leading to edema, induration, pain, and ulceration. Valvular incompetence and its clinical manifestations may also occur in the absence of clinical evidence of DVT and without the associated scarring of valves characteristic of postphlebitic incompetence. In either case, knowledge of the presence and location of incompetent venous valves is important in planning surgical treatment. DCI permits the identification of valvular competence and reflux. Venous flow is observed during normal respiration and during the Valsalva maneuver or abdominal compression. With these maneuvers a brief reversal of flow is seen in normal veins during valve closure, but with valvular incompetence the flow reversal is sustained (Fig. 5-16).

UPPER EXTREMITY VENOUS THROMBOSIS

Venous thrombosis is not limited to the lower extremities; it may occur in the jugular, subclavian, axillary, and arm veins. DCI is valuable in the noninvasive assessment of venous problems in these locations (Fig. 5-17). Criteria for the diagnosis of thrombosis are similar to those used in lower extremity examination. Knudson et al.[19] compared the results of DCI with those of venography, computed tomography (CT), and magnetic resonance imaging (MRI) for 130 extremities in 91 patient with suspected upper extremity venous thrombosis. Thrombi were present in 39 extremities. In studies with imaging correlation, the sensitivity and specificity of the DCI studies were 78 and 92 percent, respectively. DCI resulted in two false-negative diagnoses and one false-positive diagnosis of venous thrombosis of the subclavian vein. Four cases of isolated superior vena cava or proximal innominate

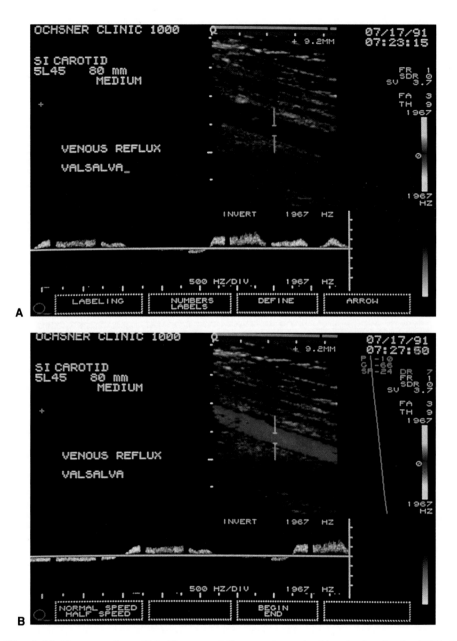

Fig. 5-16 Venous reflux. **(A)** Absence of flow at the end of inspiration in the SFV. **(B)** When a Valsalva maneuver is performed, there is sustained reversal of flow. This indicates valvular incompetence.

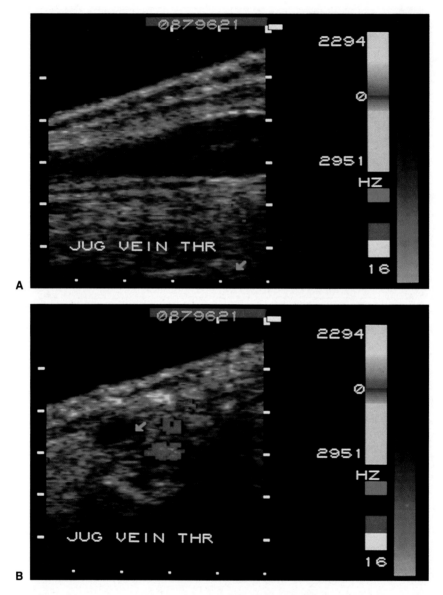

Fig. 5-17 Jugular vein thrombosis. **(A)** Longitudinal and **(B)** transverse views show the jugular vein to be distended, and DCI shows no evidence of flow. The vein was not compressible. Flow in the common carotid artery (red) is present.

vein obstruction were also missed by DCI. Although these investigators considered DCI an accurate method for the evaluation of upper extremity DVT, they emphasized the need for additional imaging tests when the DCI study is negative and central venous thrombosis is suspected.

A study by Hubsch et al.[20] of thrombosis of the internal jugular and subclavian vein caused by central venous catheters indicated that DCI was very useful. Of 26 patients with clinically suspected thrombosis, 25 were diagnosed with thrombosis of the internal jugular or subclavian vein; in addition, the degree of venous obstruction was determined and small subcutaneous collaterals were detected. Grassi and Polak[21] also used real-time ultrasonography and DCI to evaluate upper extremity venous thrombosis and compared sonographic findings with the results of conventional contrast venography in 13 patients. Absence of flow signals was noted in five patients with complete occlusion of the subclavian vein, and decreased flow signal was seen in two patients with partial obstruction of the subclavian vein. Findings returned to normal at color Doppler flow ultrasound and venography in five patients, and patent collateral veins were seen in one patient. For the initial evaluation of patients suspected of having thrombosis in the jugular, subclavian, axillary, and arm veins, we believe that DCI is an excellent choice. If DCI fails to confirm thrombosis, or the examination is technically inadequate, other imaging studies may be needed. However, in our experience this is uncommon.

OTHER NONINVASIVE TESTS

In addition to ultrasound, noninvasive means for assessment of DVT include impedance plethysmography (IPG), radionuclide venography, and iodine-125 radionuclide fibrinogen scanning. DCI has several notable advantages over IPG and radionuclide techniques. IPG is based on charges in electrical resistance at the calf that are related to the rate of venous emptying after release of a compression tourniquet. With IPG, false-positives may occur as a result of residual post-phlebitic obstruction or extrinsic venous compression as from tumor, Baker cyst, etc. Increased central venous pressure or venous compression by a pelvic mass may also result in false-positive IPG results. Likewise, false-negatives with IPG may result from nonoccluding thrombus, thrombus confined to the calf veins, and extensive venous collaterals. DCI largely avoids these pitfalls. In our experience, radionuclide venography lacks sufficient specificity to serve as a definitive diagnostic method, with extrinsic venous compression producing false positive results. Iodine-125 radionuclide fibrinogen scanning has the disadvantages that it cannot adequately image thrombus in deep pelvic vessels, it gives false-positive results when inflammation is present, and it takes at least 24 to 48 hours to complete. When DCI is compared with duplex and real-time ultrasound evaluation, its results appear to be comparable in evaluating disease in the femoral and popliteal veins and superior in the evaluation of calf vein thrombosis. Improved diagnostic confidence and the ability to readily identify partially occluding thrombosis and shortened examination are significant advantages of DCI.

SUMMARY

DCI is an excellent method for evaluation of the venous system and has several distinct advantages over other methods. One of the major benefits of DCI, particularly with the addition of capabilities to image slow-flow characteristics of veins, is the ease and rapidity of evaluating the lower extremity veins, including not only the femoral and popliteal system but also the major calf veins. The identification of nonoccluding intraluminal thrombus is enhanced by the additional contrast provided by color-flow imaging. In a similar fashion, flow imaging by scanning through the urine-filled bladder permits excellent visualization of the external iliac veins, and in thin patients the common iliac veins and distal inferior vena cava can be assessed. Thus, DCI permits a more rapid examination with increased diagnostic confidence; it may also permit a more accurate examination. The noninvasive and complication-free nature of the examination recommends it strongly as the primary test, particularly in patients with contraindications to contrast evaluation.

REFERENCES

1. Coon WW, Willis PW, Keller JB: Venous thromboembolism and other venous disease in the Tecumseh community health study. Circulation 48:839, 1973
2. Roberts HJ: Controversies and enigmas in thrombophlebitis and pulmonary embolism: perspectives on alleged overdiagnosis. Angiology 31:686, 1980
3. Hull R, Hirsh J, Sackett DL, Stoddart G: Cost effectiveness of clinical diagnosis, venography, and non-invasive testing in patients with symptomatic deep vein thrombosis. N Engl J Med 304:1561, 1981
4. Sevitt S: Venous thrombosis and pulmonary embolism: their prevention by oral anticoagulants. Am J Med 33:703, 1962
5. Lundh B, Fagher B: The clinical picture of deep vein thrombosis correlated to the frequency of pulmonary embolism. Acta Med Scand 210:353, 1981
6. Mavor GE, Galloway JMD: Ileofemoral venous thrombosis: pathological considerations and surgical management. Br J Surg 56:45, 1969
7. Raghavendra BN, Rosen RJ, Lam S, et al: Deep venous thrombosis: detection by high resolution real time ultrasonography. Radiology 152:789, 1984
8. Raghavendra BN, Horii SC, Hilton S, et al: Deep venous thrombosis: detection by probe compression of veins. J Ultrasound Med 5:89, 1986
9. Effeney DJ, Friedman MB, Gooding GAW: Ileofemoral venous thrombosis: real-time ultrasound diagnosis, normal criteria, and clinical application. Radiology 150:787, 1984
10. Meritt CRB, Wooldrige S, Bluth EI, et al: Doppler color flow imaging of deep venous thrombosis: preliminary observations: Dynamic Cardiovasc Imaging 1:268, 1988
11. Foley WD, Middleton WD, Lawson TL, et al: Color Doppler ultrasound imaging of lower-extremity venous disease: AJR 152:371, 1989
12. Baxter GM, McKechnie S, Duffy P: Colour Doppler ultrasound in deep venous thrombosis: a comparison with venography. Clin Radiol 42:32, 1990
13. Polak JF, Culter SS, O'Leary DH: Deep veins of the calf: assessment with color Doppler flow imaging. Radiology 171:481, 1989
14. Eisenberg RI: Deep venous thrombosis of the lower extremity. Choosing the optimal diagnostic modality. Radiol Rep 1:65, 1988
15. Knighton RA, Priest DL, Zwiebel WJ, et al: Techniques for color flow sonography of the lower extremity. RadioGraphics 10:775, 1990
16. Fürst G, Kuhn FP, Trappe RP, Mödder U: Diagnostik der tiefen Beinvenenthrombose. Farb-Doppler-Sonographie versus Phlebographie. ROFO 152:151, 1990
17. Rose SC, Zwiebel WJ, Nelson BD, et al: Symptomatic lower extremity deep venous thrombosis: accuracy, limitations, and role of color duplex flow imaging in diagnosis. Radiology 175:639, 1990
18. van Bemmelen PS, Bedford G, Strandness DE: Visualization of calf veins by color flow imaging. Ultrasound Med Biol 16:15, 1990
19. Knudson GJ, Wiedmeyer DA, Erickson SJ, et al: Color Doppler sonographic imaging in the assessment of upper-extremity deep venous thrombosis. AJR 154:399, 1990
20. Hubsch PJ, Stiglbauer RL, Schwaighofer BW, et al: Internal jugular and subclavian vein thrombosis caused by central venous catheters. Evaluation using Doppler blood flow imaging. J Ultrasound Med 7:629, 1988
21. Grassi CJ, Polak JF: Axillary and subclavian venous thrombosis: follow-up evaluation with color Doppler flow US and venography. Radiology 175:651, 1990

6

Abdomen

Christopher R. B. Merritt

Real-time ultrasound examination of the abdomen has emphasized evaluation of morphologic changes in organ size, shape, position, contour, and parenchymal patterns. Relatively limited attention has been directed to the evaluation of abdominal vessels and organ blood flow. With B-mode gray-scale ultrasound, large vessels such as the aorta, the inferior vena cava (IVC), and the mesenteric, portal, splenic, hepatic, and renal vessels are readily identified. Although the vessel wall and lumen are seen, real-time imaging provides little if any information about flow, and significant abnormalities related to vascular thrombosis, narrowing, or changes in flow direction or dynamics may be overlooked. Duplex Doppler and Doppler color imaging (DCI) have resulted in a significant extension of the role of ultrasound in examining the abdomen, allowing determination of the presence and direction of flow along with more subtle information related to flow velocity and organ perfusion. The addition of information related to organ blood supply and organ perfusion, which is available with duplex and color Doppler instrumentation, is beginning to have a profound impact on the sonographic evaluation of the abdomen, increasing the role and range of applications of ultrasound.

As in peripheral vascular applications, DCI is not a replacement for analysis of the Doppler spectrum. DCI should be viewed as a tool to be used in conjunction with high-resolution imaging and spectral analysis. A combination of tissue and flow imaging supplemented with quantitative assessment by both DCI and duplex Doppler is an extremely powerful diagnostic combination, particularly when the speed, ease, and relatively low cost are considered.

Prior to discussion of specific uses of DCI in the abdomen, it is necessary to point out that quality ultrasonography, be it imaging, duplex Doppler, or DCI, demands special skills in the operation of equipment as well as training and experience in the interpretation of the results. The successful interpretation of a DCI examination requires an understanding of the basic principles and the unique nature of the Doppler information, as well as knowledge of the techniques and instrumentation necessary to ensure the generation of high-quality data. Also needed is a knowledge of the patterns of normal and abnormal flow necessary to establish a diagnosis. The operator must monitor the quality of the data generated in the examination and differentiate real and clinically important findings from artifact. This is particularly true for the abdomen, where greater examination depths result in the potential for artifacts and technical errors not usually encountered in peripheral vascular applications. Serious pitfalls await the careless or poorly trained user, no matter how sophisticated the machine being used, and ultimately the success or failure of the investigation is determined by clinical, technical, and interpretive skill and not by the machine.[1]

OVERVIEW OF ABDOMINAL APPLICATIONS

The most important applications of DCI in the abdomen are

Differentiation of vascular from nonvascular structures

Identification of vessels

Mapping of vessels for duplex sampling

Determination of the direction of blood flow

Detection of vessel narrowing or occlusion

Identification of collateral vessels

Detection of arteriovenous malformations

Diagnosis of aneurysm and pseudoaneurysm

Characterization of flow to organs

Evaluation of transplant vascular supply

Characterization of malignant tumors

These applications include identification of vessels, determination of the direction of blood flow, detection and measurement of vessel narrowing or occlusion, characterization of flow to organs and tumors, and mapping of vessels not visible on conventional images for duplex sampling. In addition to the obvious use of DCI in identification of occlusion, stenosis, and flow disturbances in major vessels, duplex and color Doppler information is of growing importance in inference of abnormalities in the peripheral vascular bed of an organ or tissue. Changes in the spectral waveform or (for DCI) in the appearance of flow in diastole

provide insight into the resistance of the vascular bed supplied by the vessel and, although not specific, may indicate changes due to a variety of conditions including transplant rejection, acute inflammation, and malignant tumors.

Guided by DCI, Doppler spectral analysis of flow in large vessels supplying the liver, kidneys, or mesentery may be used to infer the presence and severity of proximal stenosis. Large-vessel changes (such as flow reversal in the portal vein, the presence of portosystemic collaterals, and the occlusion of portal, splenic, or renal veins) and mesenteric or renal artery stenosis are all identifiable by Doppler ultrasonographic methods. Changes in distal vascular impedance may also be inferred from the Doppler spectrum and in some cases from the DCI examination.[2] In the evaluation of small-vessel changes, DCI is of particular value because it permits rapid identification of vessels too small to be detected by conventional imaging equipment, thus permitting more accurate sampling for duplex Doppler spectral analysis. Doppler changes reflecting abnormal impedance of the vascular bed may also be important in the early identification of rejection of transplanted organs and may aid in differentiation of benign and malignant masses. It is accepted that changes in tissue function are often associated with changes in blood flow, and duplex Doppler ultrasound and DCI, with their abilities to display such changes, are leading us closer to the long-sought goal of noninvasive tissue characterization.[3-5]

LIVER

The liver is the best suited of all of the abdominal organs for ultrasound examination. Complete ultrasound evaluation of the liver should be based on a systematic assessment of hepatic size, position, contour, and parenchyma and of the hepatic vessels. The generally homogeneous sonographic appearance of the hepatic parenchyma makes the identification of focal abnormalities relatively straightforward and aids in the imaging of the hepatic and portal veins and their major branches. The importance of careful inspection of the hepatic vasculature in the identification of hepatic abnormalities has not been adequately emphasized in most discussions of hepatic ultrasonography. The real-time imaging of hepatic vasculature permits the identification of thrombosis of the portal vein,[6,7] vascular displacement,[8] intravascular gas,[9] and development of collateral circulation in portal hypertension. Normal vascular anatomy and anatomic variations involving vessels in the porta hepatis can be rapidly evaluated by DCI to differentiate vascular structures. Also, the ability of DCI to distinguish vascular from nonvascular structures allows quick and accurate differentiation of an enlarged hepatic artery from the bile duct; in view of the relatively common incidence of anatomic variation in the relationships of the vessels in the portal triad, this is often useful. Not only do the hepatic and portal vessels provide clues to hepatic pathology, but also they provide anatomic landmarks essential for accurate localization of intrahepatic lesions. DCI may serve as an extremely useful adjunct to real-time imaging in the identification and evaluation of these important landmarks, especially when the vessels are small or compressed by hepatic disease.

The first requirement for evaluation of the hepatic vasculature, whether by ultrasound imaging alone, DCI, or duplex Doppler, is an understanding of hepatic vascular anatomy and its normal sonographic appearance. The liver is a bilobed organ that begins as a bud from the foregut and, during development, branches into a series of divisions that form the hepatic segments. The segmental anatomy of the liver is reflected in the distribution of major blood vessels (Figs. 6-1 and 6-2).[10] The hepatic veins lie at the bound-

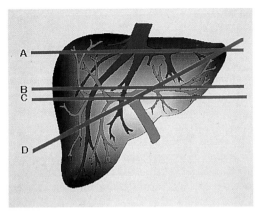

Fig. 6-1 Hepatic vascular anatomy. The hepatic veins (dark blue) and portal veins (light blue) serve as landmarks for evaluation of hepatic segmental anatomy. Levels for the transverse sections shown in Figures 6-2A to D are indicated.

aries of the hepatic segments, whereas the portal veins and hepatic arteries are located in the central portions of the hepatic segments. The interlobar fissure is defined by the plane of the middle hepatic vein. The left hepatic vein separates the medial and lateral segments of the left lobe, and the right hepatic vein separates the anterior and posterior segments of the right lobe. The anterior and posterior segmental branches of the right portal vein are located centrally within their respective hepatic segments, and the right hepatic vein divides these segments. The anterior and posterior segmental branches of the right portal vein supply the anterior and posterior segments of the right hepatic lobe. The plane separating the medial and lateral segments of the left lobe is indicated by the location of the ligamentum teres hepatis. The interlobar fissure is along a plane defined by the gallbladder fossa and the middle hepatic vein.

Examination Technique

DCI, duplex Doppler, and ultrasound imaging of the liver and its vessels require frequencies of 2.25 to 5.0 MHz, depending on

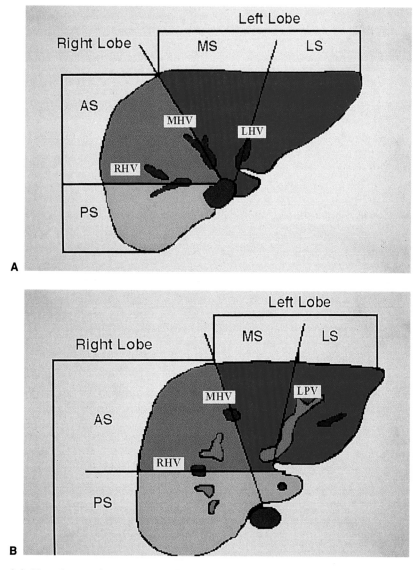

Fig. 6-2 Hepatic vascular anatomy. **(A–D)** Transverse sections corresponding to the levels indicated in Figure 6-1 show the relationship of hepatic veins (dark blue) and portal veins (light blue) to the lobar and segmental boundaries of the liver. (*Figure continues.*)

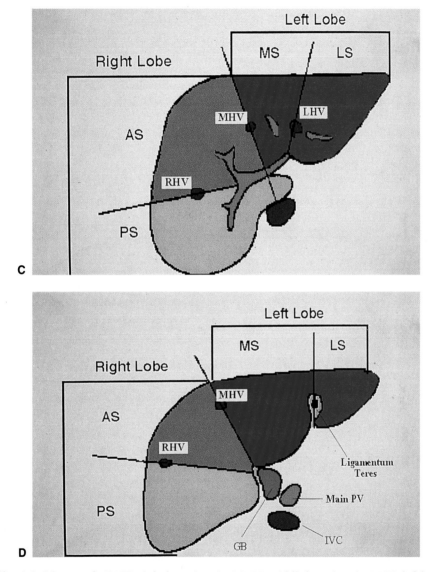

Fig. 6-2 (*Continued*). RHV, right hepatic vein; MHV, middle hepatic vein; LHV, left hepatic vein; Main PV, main portal vein; LPV, left portal vein; AS, anterior segment right hepatic lobe; PS, posterior segment right hepatic lobe; MS, medial segment left hepatic lobe; LS, lateral segment left hepatic lobe; GB, gallbladder.

the size of the patient and the depth of the vessel to be examined. To obtain the maximal signal from the vessel of interest, the examiner must make every effort to reduce the Doppler angle as much as possible. This is particularly true when low-velocity flow in deep venous structures is being evaluated. A systematic inspection of hepatic vascular landmarks by DCI should include the following:

1. Patency of the main, right, and left portal veins should be confirmed. Flow should also be identified in the anterior and posterior segmental branches of the right portal vein and the medial and lateral segments of the left portal vein.

2. The diameter of the portal vein should be noted, as a diameter greater than 12 mm suggests portal hypertension. DCI and, if necessary, duplex Doppler may be used to determine whether flow is hepatopedal or hepatofugal.

3. The left, middle, and right hepatic veins should be visualized. Normally these vessels have a straight and regular course, and irregularities or deviations should be noted because they often indicate parenchymal disease or the presence of a mass. DCI is particularly helpful in visualization of the smaller and more peripheral branches of these vessels.

4. The IVC should be evaluated for patency, narrowing or extrinsic compression, or displacement by hepatic or retrocaval masses.

5. The area of the ligamentum teres should be examined for evidence of paraumbilical collaterals. DCI is especially helpful in this assessment since small portosystemic collaterals developing along the course of the ligamentum teres and umbilical vein are often visible by DCI before they become obvious by imaging alone.

6. If a mass is present, its relationship to the hepatic and portal veins should be carefully mapped out and the segment(s) occupied by the mass clearly specified in the report.

Hepatic Vascular Abnormalities

Vascular abnormalities visible by ultrasound may result from extrinsic causes producing vessel compression, displacement, encasement, or changes in relative wall echogenicity. Ultrasound may also demonstrate intrinsic abnormalities including tumor, thrombus, aneurysm, dilatation, and intraluminal gas. Each of these abnormalities may be the only manifestation of hepatic abnormality resulting from a wide range of causes, including primary and secondary malignant tumors, diffuse infiltration, and inflammatory diseases.

Inferior Vena Cava and Hepatic Veins

NORMAL

The IVC and the main left, middle, and right hepatic veins are normally visible by DCI. The display of flow in the IVC by using DCI is made difficult by the deep location of the vessel and problems in obtaining an acceptable Doppler angle for measurement of flow. Since the course of the IVC is generally parallel to the skin surface, sagittal, parasagittal, and coronal imaging planes result in Doppler angles approaching 90 degrees unless beam steering or wedges are used to reduce the angle of the beam to the direction of flow.

The hepatic veins all communicate with the IVC, and none has a significant extrahepatic course. The main left and right hepatic veins drain directly into the IVC. The middle hepatic vein may drain into the left hepatic vein or directly into the IVC. In addition to the three main hepatic veins, up to 12 to 15 smaller hepatic venous branches may directly enter the IVC from the posterior aspect of the right hepatic lobe. Detection of flow in the hepatic veins is considerably easier than in the IVC because the hepatic veins radiate from the periphery of the liver toward the IVC and flow more or less away from the transducer with a small Doppler angle. Transverse images in the subxiphoid region provide excellent views of the left hepatic vein and its junction with the IVC (Fig. 6-3A). Transverse subcostal or oblique images through the rib cage from a more lateral approach permit imaging of the middle and right hepatic veins (Fig. 6-3B). Longitudinal images of these vessels may be similarly obtained (Fig. 6-3C and D). As with other ultrasound imaging approaches, the examination technique should be optimized for each patient. A selection of linear, convex, and phased arrays of frequencies from 2.25 to 5.0 MHz is valuable and permits the examiner to select the optimal transducer on the basis of patient size, liver size and location, and configuration of the rib cage.

The flow dynamics in the hepatic veins and IVC are complex compared with venous waveforms encountered elsewhere in the abdomen. Doppler spectra obtained from the IVC and normal hepatic veins are similar and have a phasic flow pattern. Flow varies with changes in respiration, abdominal pressure, and right atrial pressure. Since there are no functional valves between the IVC, the hepatic veins, and the right atrium, variations in flow related to cardiac pulsation are transmitted directly to these vessels. During atrial systole a rapid reversal of flow due to regurgitation of blood from the right atrium is noted, with antegrade flow in diastole (Fig. 6-4).

Respiration also affects flow velocity in the hepatic veins and IVC. There is diminished flow when intrathoracic pressure is increased or intra-abdominal pressure is reduced. These conditions are seen at the end of inspiration or during a Valsalva maneuver. Conversely, flow velocity in these vessels increases when intrathoracic pressure is reduced and abdominal pressure is increased. For example, during inspiration there is decreased intrathoracic pressure and increased intra-abdominal pressure, causing increased flow toward the heart. These dynamics are reversed during expiration. In most persons, at the end of inspiration (which is when most patients are asked to suspend respiration for

scanning) there is an increase in thoracic pressure (a Valsalva) and flow diminishes or stops. This makes the collection of Doppler information from the hepatic veins and IVC difficult during breath holding. The ability of DCI to provide a continuous display of flow overcomes this disadvantage and permits easy inspection of the dynamics of hepatic vein and IVC flow under the influence of normal respiration and artificial changes in thoracic or abdominal pressure performed to augment flow and increase vessel visibility.

ABNORMAL

The major abnormalities affecting the IVC and hepatic veins are thrombosis and compression or occlusion due to space-occupying disease. Most often this is the result of diffuse hepatic parenchymal disease such as cirrhosis. In these patients compression of normal hepatic veins may make evaluation by real-time imaging extremely difficult, if not impossible. DCI generally permits visualization of compressed hepatic veins that are not identifiable by conventional imaging (Fig. 6-5). Hepatic venous outflow obstruction may result from microscopic veno-occlusive disease affecting the centrilobular venous radicals or from obstruction of major hepatic veins as they approach or enter the IVC. Hepatic veno-occlusive disease due to thrombosis as part of the Budd-Chiari syndrome is relatively uncommon. In the Budd-Chiari syndrome, hepatic venous outflow obstruction may result from obstruction of the hepatic vein or IVC by tumor, by venous thrombosis secondary to myeloproliferative disease, or as a result of a fibrous diaphragm or web just above the entrance of the left and middle hepatic veins. Before the introduction of DCI, duplex Doppler was used in the sonographic evaluation of patients with Budd-Chiari syndrome, and it generally correlated well with therapeutic results and angiographic findings. Pulsed-Doppler sonography in Budd-Chiari syndrome reveals absent blood flow in the IVC and hepatic veins or

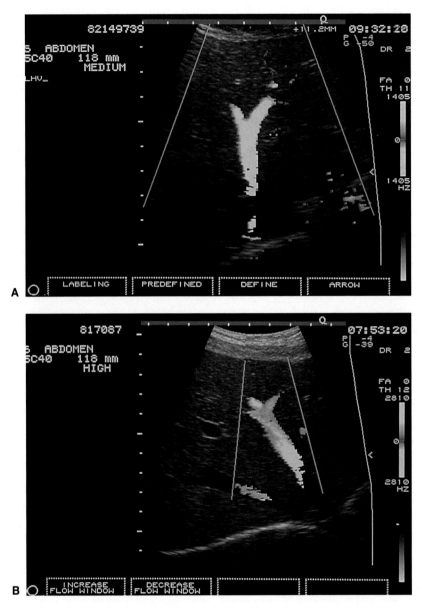

Fig. 6-3 Normal hepatic veins. **(A)** Transverse subxiphoid image shows the left hepatic vein as it approaches the IVC. The middle and right hepatic veins are shown without flow because of a suboptimal Doppler angle. **(B)** Subcostal transverse image shows the middle and right hepatic veins. The flow shown in the middle hepatic vein (MHV) is less saturated than that in the right hepatic vein (RHV). This does not indicate higher velocity in the MHV, but is a result of a larger Doppler angle for the RHV than for the MHV. (*Figure continues.*)

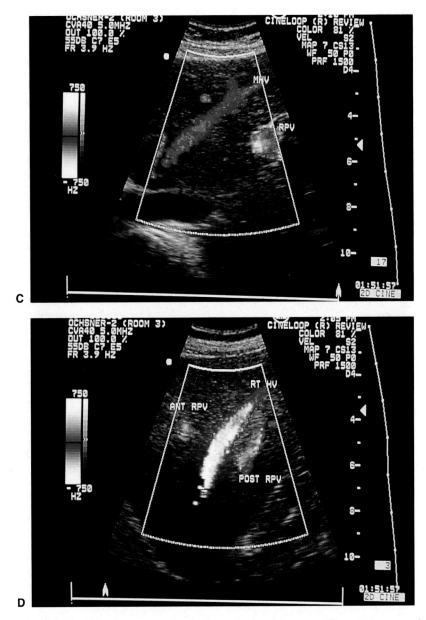

Fig. 6-3 (*Continued*). **(C)** Longitudinal image shows the MHV (blue) as it approaches the IVC. Note the relationship of the MHV as it passes anterior to the right portal vein (RPV) (red). The red vessel anterior to the MHV is a part of the medial segmental branch of the left portal vein (LPV). **(D)** Longitudinal image of RHV. Note the position of the RHV as it passes midway between the anterior and posterior segmental branches of the RPV and delineates the boundary between the anterior and posterior segments of the right lobe.

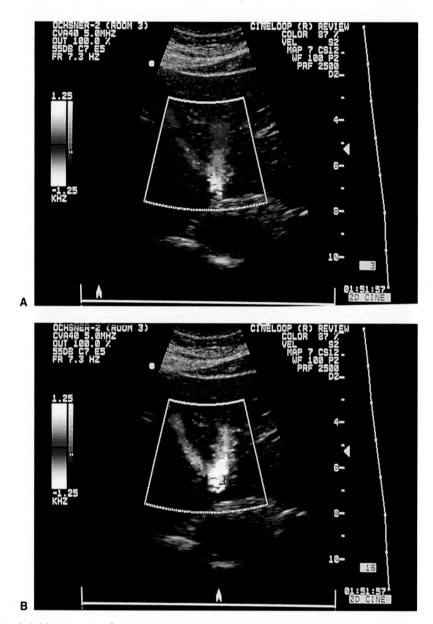

Fig. 6-4 Hepatic vein flow. **(A)** Images of the left and middle hepatic vein during atrial diastole show flow from the liver into the IVC (blue). **(B)** With systolic contraction of the right atrium, there is brief flow reversal in the vein (red). (*Figure continues.*)

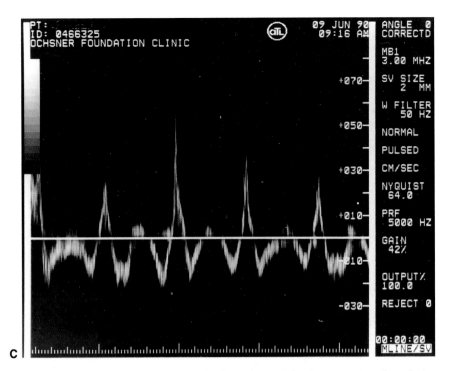

Fig. 6-4 (*Continued*). **(C)** Spectral Doppler from the IVC has better temporal resolution and shows these variations in more detail.

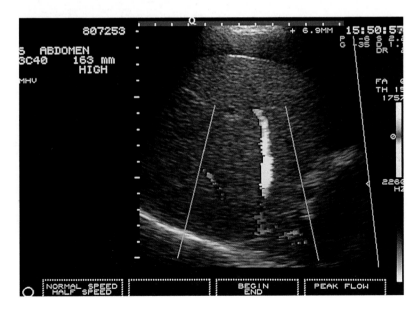

Fig. 6-5 Right hepatic vein. Transverse image of the right hepatic lobe in a patient with cirrhosis and ascites shows the right hepatic vein clearly. With gray-scale imaging alone, the vessel was not visible.

Portal Vein

NORMAL

The portal vein drains the splanchnic circulation and carries about 75 percent of the afferent flow to the liver. The formation of the main portal vein by the junction of the splenic and superior mesenteric veins posterior to the neck of the pancreas is regularly seen by DCI (Fig. 6-7). Usually the main portal vein lies posterior to both the bile duct and the hepatic artery as it passes to the right in the free edge of the lesser omentum (Fig. 6-8). At the hilum of the liver the main portal vein divides into main branches to the right and left hepatic lobes. As shown in Figure 6-1, the portal vein has a regular pattern of branching within the liver. Unlike for the hepatic artery, major abnormalities in the branching pattern of the portal vein are rare. The right portal vein is usually shorter than 3 cm,[16] dividing into anterior and posterior branches. Each branch has superior and inferior divisions, each supplying a different hepatic segment. The left portal vein is directed anteriorly and to the left, dividing into medial and lateral branches. The left portal vein is joined by the ligamentum teres (the obliterated umbilical vein) near its bifurcation into medial and lateral divisions. This is an important anatomic reference site because the junction of the ligamentum teres and the left portal vein marks the location of paraumbilical portosystemic collaterals common in patients with portal hypertension. This area should always be carefully evaluated by DCI, particularly in patients with cirrhosis.

Subcostal and transhepatic approaches with 2.25- to 5.0-MHz transducers are usually required for DCI evaluation of the intrahepatic and extrahepatic portions of the portal vein. Because of the limitations for access posed

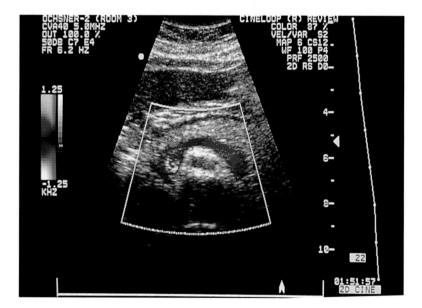

Fig. 6-7 Normal portal vein. Transverse image at the level of the pancreas shows the confluence of the splenic vein (red) and mesenteric vein (blue) to form the portal vein. The change in color of flow in the splenic vein as it passes over the SMA is an indication of a change in the direction of flow with respect to the transducer.

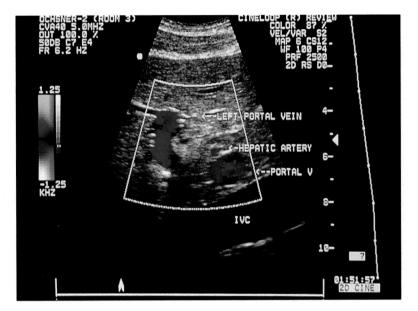

Fig. 6-8 Normal main and left portal veins. Longitudinal parasagittal image shows the main portal vein as it passes anterior to the IVC. Here the portal vein (blue) most often lies posterior to the hepatic artery (red) and bile duct (not shown). The left portal vein (red) is also shown passing anteriorly into the left lobe of the liver. The difference in color of the main portal vein and the hepatic artery suggests hepatofugal portal vein flow; however, additional images showed this to be due to tortuosity of the hepatic artery.

by the rib cage, acoustic windows for DCI of the portal vein should be selected carefully, keeping in mind the expected course of the vessel of interest and the necessity of maintaining a relatively small Doppler angle to maximize the Doppler frequency shift detected. Since the left portal vein is directed anteriorly, it is usually seen well in parasagittal and longitudinal images obtained by scanning through the left lobe of the liver with the transducer positioned in the subxiphoid space (Fig. 6-8). This results in a small Doppler angle and increases the detectability of flow signal, permitting rapid determination of the presence and direction of flow. Unfortunately, this access site is highly unsuitable for evaluation of the main and right portal veins because these vessels flow at almost 90 degrees to the insonating beam. Angulation of the transducer to the right is often of minimal value because the course of the

anterior segmental branch of the hepatic artery and portal vein maintains an unfavorable Doppler angle. Attention to the Doppler angle is particularly important in obtaining measurements from the right portal vein, because the use of a large (>60-degree) angle may make it difficult to detect flow and can also result in an ambiguous display of flow direction. The best approach for evaluation of flow in the right portal vein and its main branches is to scan through an intercostal space with the ultrasound beam angled medially. If the liver extends beneath the costal margin, a subcostal approach in the sagittal plane with medial angulation of the transducer may also provide a good look at these vessels.

Duplex Doppler of the main portal vein reveals a continuous flow pattern with variations in velocity induced by respiration. In

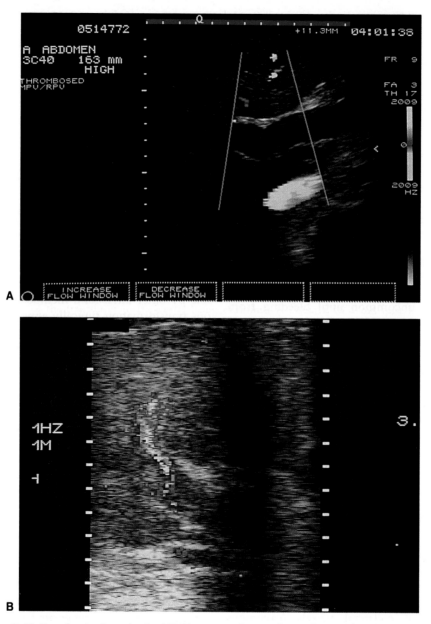

Fig. 6-10 Portal vein thrombosis. **(A)** Transverse image shows flow within the IVC (blue), but no flow is present in the portal vein as it passes anterior to the IVC. Faint echoes are present within the portal vein, indicating thrombosis. Care should be taken in interpreting the DCI findings in this image because the Doppler angle is nearly 90 degrees to the direction of flow in the portal vein. **(B)** Longitudinal view of the right portal vein shows absence of flow from the proximal portion of the right portal due to thrombosis. More distally within the portal vein, hepatopedal flow (blue) is seen. This is provided by collaterals that bypass the obstructed segment. (Fig. B from Merritt,[20] with permission.)

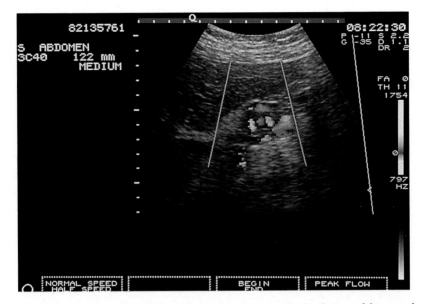

```
82135761                              08:22:30
                                      P -11  S 2.2
S  ABDOMEN                            G -35  D T.1
3C40    122 mm                              DR   2
        MEDIUM
                                           FA   0
                                           TH  11
                                              1754

                                              0

                                              797
                                              HZ

NORMAL SPEED          BEGIN      PEAK FLOW
HALF SPEED            END
```

Fig. 6-11 Cavernous transformation of the portal vein. Longitudinal view of the porta hepatis in a patient with portal vein thrombosis shows numerous vascular structures in the region of the portal vein. Spectral Doppler confirmed venous waveforms. The color arises from flow in numerous portal collateral veins.

ditis. Intrahepatic portal hypertension may result from alcoholic cirrhosis, chronic active hepatitis, and primary biliary cirrhosis. Less common causes include hemochromatosis and cirrhosis associated with Wilson's disease, secondary biliary cirrhosis, and α_1-antitrypsin deficiency. Extrahepatic portal vein obstruction is typically due to portal vein thrombosis or obstruction by tumor. Regardless of the cause, the primary change present in portal hypertension is the development of collateral circulation to bypass the obstructed portal veins. Once the pressure in the portal vein exceeds about 10 mmHg, collateral vessels develop between the high-pressure portal vessels and low-pressure systemic veins. Numerous potential collateral pathways exist, and many are demonstrable by DCI.

In patients with portal hypertension DCI allows rapid determination of the direction of portal blood flow (Fig. 6-13). This infor-

mation is important in planning surgical treatment because the presence of hepatofugal flow indicates the need for a portocaval or mesocaval rather than a splenorenal shunt. Paraumbilical, gastroesophageal, pancreaticoduodenal, retroperitoneal, splenorenal, and gastrorenal collaterals have all been described by using duplex or DCI methods. DCI often indicates the presence of more extensive collaterals than suggested by grayscale imaging alone (Fig. 6-14). In all patients with chronic liver disease or portal hypertension, any unusual tubular structure in the abdomen should be evaluated by Doppler, since many of these will turn out to be collateral veins decompressing the obstructed portal venous system. Shunting of blood into these collaterals may be seen with preservation of hepatopedal flow in the main portal vein branches or, less commonly, with hepatofugal portal vein flow. Flow direction in patients with portosystemic collaterals through the paraumbilical veins should be

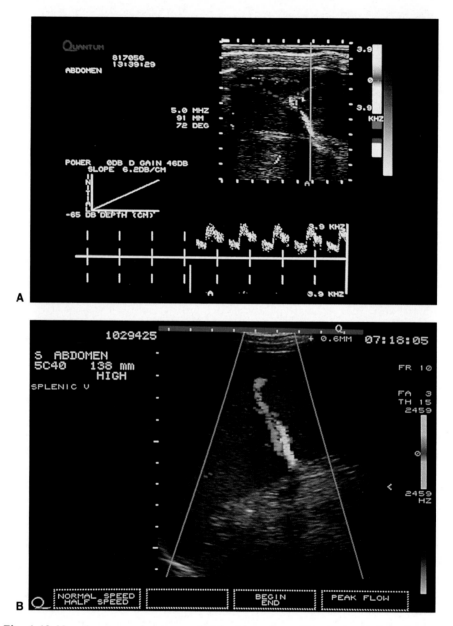

Fig. 6-12 Hepatic artery enlargement. **(A)** In this patient with portal vein thrombosis, characteristic enlargement of the hepatic artery is seen. **(B)** Hepatic artery enlargement (red vessel) is seen in a patient with portal hypertension and reversed portal vein flow (blue vessel). In patients with cirrhosis or portal vein thrombosis and jaundice, DCI is useful in differentiation of hepatic artery dilatation from bile duct enlargement.

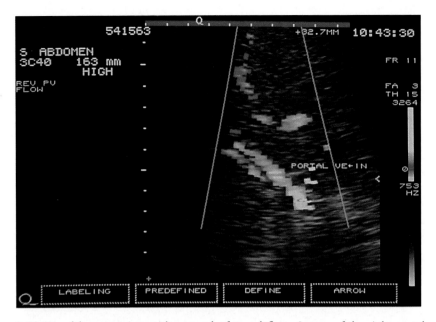

Fig. 6-13 Portal hypertension with reversal of portal flow. Image of the right portal vein shows flow away from the transducer in the portal vein (blue), while flow direction in the accompanying hepatic artery (red) is normal. The hepatic artery is enlarged.

evaluated with care. Flow through these collaterals is from the left portal vein where it joins the ligamentum teres hepatis. In patients with portal hypertension it is possible to see hepatopedal flow in the left portal vein with hepatofugal flow in the right portal vein. This is because blood from the right portal vein is redirected through the ascending segment of the left portal vein to the umbilical collateral, resulting in normal flow direction in the main portion of the left portal vein.

Portosystemic shunts may develop spontaneously through collateral vessels or may be created surgically to treat symptomatic portal hypertension. DCI is valuable in confirming the patency of surgically created portosystemic shunts from the portal or mesenteric vein to the IVC (portocaval and mesocaval shunts), from the splenic vein to the renal vein (distal splenorenal or Warren shunts), or from the mesenteric vein to the right atrium (mesoatrial shunt), provided that an adequate acoustic window is available. The patency of portocaval shunts is determined by the demonstration of flow from the portal vein into the IVC, often with direct visualization of the portal vein–to–IVC anastomosis (Fig. 6-15). In splenorenal shunts, patency is established by demonstration of flow in both the splenic and renal veins in appropriate directions. Ralls et al.[23] have reported success with DCI in demonstrating portocaval shunt patency in eight of nine patients, and Grant et al.[15] have reported successful inference of shunt patency or thrombosis in 100 percent of 22 portosystemic shunts correlated with angiography or MRI. In the evaluation of 32 shunts, the anasto-

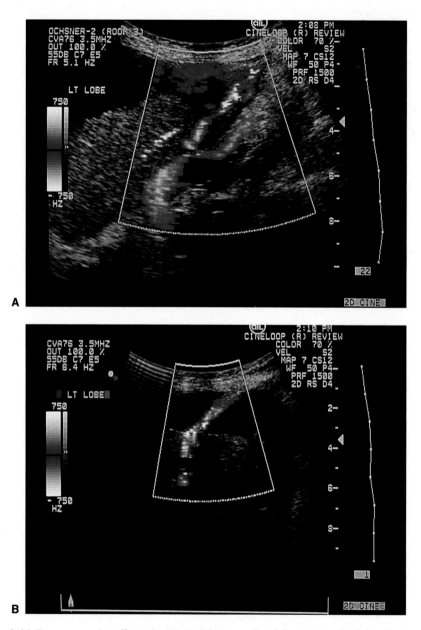

Fig. 6-14 Portosystemic collaterals. **(A & B)** Hepatofugal flow from the left portal vein is seen along the ligamentum teres hepatis and falciform ligament in a patient with portal hypertension. (*Figure continues.*)

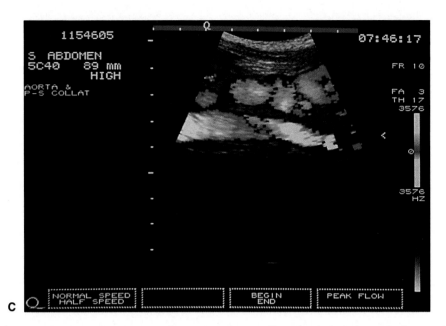

Fig. 6-14 (*Continued*). **(C)** In another patient, large collateral veins are shown in the anterior abdominal wall near the midline.

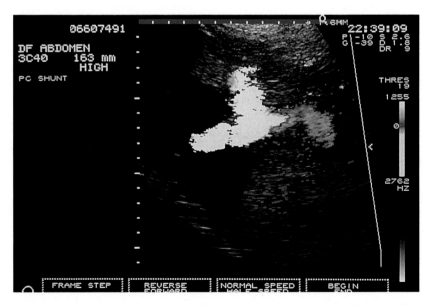

Fig. 6-15 Portacaval shunt. Longitudinal view shows a patent portacaval shunt. The communication between the portal vein and IVC is widely patent, and the color (blue) indicates that the direction of flow is from the portal vein into the IVC.

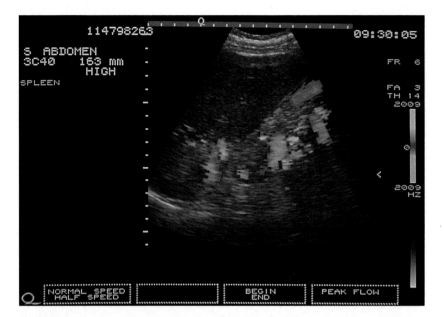

Fig. 6-16 Splenorenal collaterals. Images of the region of the splenic hilum and left kidney reveal numerous vascular structures in a patient with portal hypertension. With real-time imaging, splenic to left renal vein collaterals could be traced. The findings indicate a spontaneous splenorenal shunt. DCI is also useful in monitoring the patency of surgically created splenorenal shunts.

mosis was shown clearly by DCI in 23, probably in 4, and not all in 5. Although duplex Doppler and DCI were similar in establishing patency in portacaval, mesocaval, and mesoatrial shunts, DCI was clearly superior in the evaluation of splenorenal shunts. In patients with splenorenal shunts, scanning through the spleen usually allows good visualization of the vessels of interest (Fig. 6-16). Mesoatrial shunts are used to treat hepatic vein occlusion and consist of a synthetic graft from the mesenteric vein to the right atrium. These grafts are usually placed anterior to the liver and therefore are quite superficial, making sonographic evaluation relatively easy. Patency is confirmed by the identification of flow toward the heart anywhere along the course of the graft.

Other Portal Vein Changes

Portal vein aneurysms are uncommon findings arising from anomalous communica-tions between the portal and hepatic veins and resulting in shunting of flow from the portal to the hepatic venous system.[5,24] Small shunts from the portal vein to the hepatic vein may occur in patients with cirrhosis, but larger vascular malformations are rare and are thought to arise congenitally or to result from trauma. DCI is ideally suited for the identification of these unusual vessels and reveals turbulent flow in the aneurysm along with the dilated vessels associated with the lesion (Fig. 6-17).

Hepatic Artery

The normal hepatic artery lies along the portal vein. Its evaluation by DCI is similar to evaluation of the portal vein. Axial or sagittal imaging planes in the epigastrium and subxiphoid region permit interrogation of the origin of the hepatic artery from the celiac axis or, in the case of anomaly, from the superior mesenteric artery. There is considerable

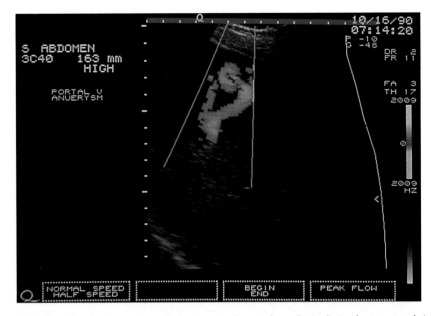

Fig. 6-17 Portal vein aneurysm. A large portal vein branch (red) is shown supplying a rounded vascular structure (blue) in the right hepatic lobe. Additional views showed a large hepatic vein draining this structure. The lesion is caused by an anomalous connection between the portal and hepatic veins, forming a portal vein aneurysm.

variation in the relationship of the intrahepatic branches of the hepatic artery relative to the portal vein and bile duct. Most often, the main hepatic artery lies anterior and to the left of the portal vein, next to the bile duct. At the level of the hepatoduodenal ligament, the hepatic artery usually lies between the portal vein and the bile duct, although in about 15 percent of patients it lies anterior to the bile duct. Within the liver the usual location is also between the portal vein and the bile duct; however, in 10 to 15 percent of patients it is anterior to, and in 5 to 10 percent it is posterior to, the portal vein.[25] The intrahepatic portions of the hepatic artery along the portal vein are usually best evaluated by using intercostal or subcostal acoustic windows scanning through the liver (Fig. 6-18). DCI is particularly helpful in identifying the presence and location of the hepatic artery for Doppler sampling in hepatic transplant recipients. The normal hepatic artery has a low-impedance Doppler waveform with continuous diastolic flow, features that are better visualized by spectral analysis than by DCI.

Perhaps the most common and useful application of DCI of the hepatic artery is in quickly differentiating vascular and avascular tubular structures in the porta hepatis, since anatomic variants in this region are relatively common. Frequently the hepatic artery is as large as or larger than the bile duct, giving rise to possible confusion and misdiagnosis, which are easily resolved by the use of DCI (Fig. 6-19).[26] DCI also permits identification of flow redistribution between the portal venous and hepatic arterial systems in patients with portal hypertension.[27] Abnormalities of hepatic artery anatomy are relatively common, and angiography is generally regarded as definitive. Ultrasound is effective in the identification of replaced hepatic arteries, with a sensitivity of 71 percent and a specificity of 96 percent reported by Bret et al.[28]

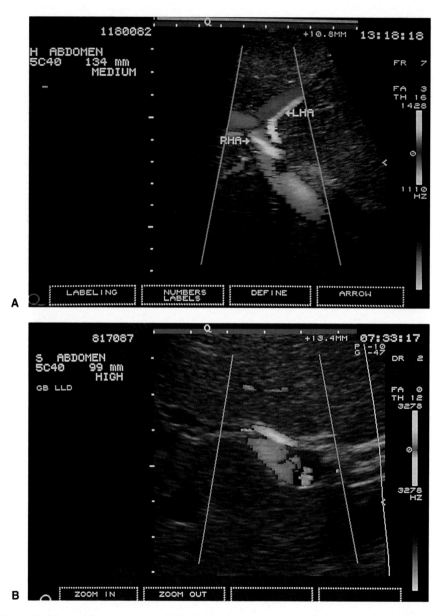

Fig. 6-18 Normal hepatic artery. **(A)** The higher velocities in the hepatic artery than in the portal vein permit differentiation of these vessels despite their proximity and their similar flow direction. With some DCI instruments, velocities above a certain threshold may be tagged with a special color, permitting areas of high velocity to be quickly differentiated. RHA, right hepatic artery; LHA, left hepatic artery. **(B)** The normal display is shown. (*Figure continues.*)

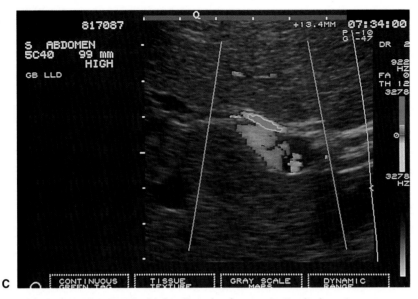

Fig. 6-18 (*Continued*). **(C)** The higher Doppler frequencies in the hepatic artery are tagged in green, allowing easy differentiation from the lower frequencies in the portal vein (red).

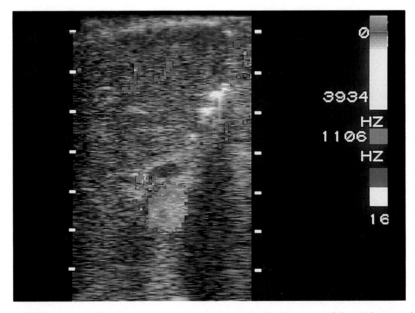

Fig. 6-19 Bile duct and normal hepatic artery. Longitudinal image of the right portal vein shows the hepatic artery (green) anterior to the portal vein. The adjacent bile duct shows no flow and is easily differentiated from the hepatic artery.

DCI could reasonably be expected to offer comparable or better results. Aneurysms of the hepatic artery are uncommon and may arise from arteriosclerosis or be secondary to trauma.[29] Several reports of the successful use of duplex ultrasound to evaluate these conditions have appeared in the literature.[30] DCI should be of equal or greater efficacy in evaluating these conditions.

Hepatic Transplantation

Doppler ultrasound is critical in both the pre- and postoperative assessment of hepatic transplant recipients. Most published studies dealing with the role of Doppler in patients receiving liver transplants have emphasized duplex Doppler. Our experience indicates that DCI is an extremely useful adjunct to duplex Doppler in the evaluation of hepatic blood flow both before and after transplantation. DCI does not replace the need for careful sampling and analysis of the Doppler spectrum, but it does significantly improve the speed and efficiency of examination.

Also, the confidence of diagnoses of arterial or venous occlusion is improved by using DCI as well as duplex ultrasound in the postoperative setting. Before transplantation, the anatomy and patency of the IVC, hepatic veins, and portal veins must be confirmed (Fig. 6-20). In children with biliary atresia, identification of common anatomic variants of the IVC and hepatic vessels is facilitated by using Doppler, particularly DCI. After transplantation, Doppler methods are essential to confirm hepatic arterial and portal venous patency, especially in the early postoperative period, when the risk of thrombosis is greatest (Fig. 6-21). Loss of hepatic arterial flow in the early post-transplant period indicates possible arterial thrombosis. Since hepatic artery thrombosis after liver transplantation is difficult to detect clinically in its early stages and is a devastating event, early identification of this complication by using Doppler may allow thrombectomy rather than retransplantation. Duplex sonography is highly sensitive in detecting hepatic artery thrombosis after liver transplan-

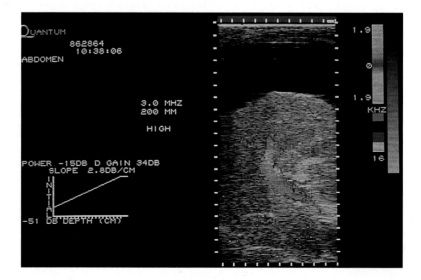

Fig. 6-20 Before liver transplantation. Longitudinal image shows a shrunken cirrhotic liver surrounded by ascites. The main portal vein (blue) is patent and exhibits hepatopedal flow.

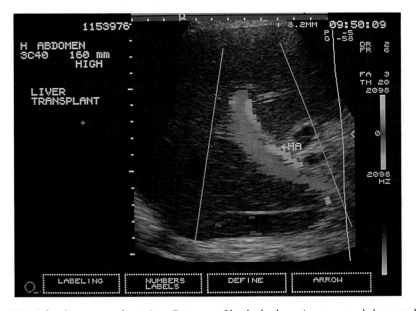

Fig. 6-21 After liver transplantation. Patency of both the hepatic artery and the portal vein is indicated by DCI in longitudinal image of the right hepatic lobe of a liver transplant recipient.

tation, and Doppler of the hepatic artery combined with real-time sonography of the liver parenchyma is regarded as the optimal procedure for selecting patients who require hepatic angiography after liver transplantation.[31,32] Doppler ultrasonography is also useful in monitoring the response to intraarterial thrombolytic treatment for hepatic artery thrombosis following liver transplantation.[33] Again, the addition of DCI would appear to offer valuable benefits. The role of Doppler in the diagnosis of hepatic transplant rejection is less well established, although changes in the hepatic arterial resistive index (RI) have been suggested as indicating graft dysfunction in some studies.[34,35] It should be noted that rejection in the absence of Doppler waveform abnormalities may also occur. DCI would appear to have a relatively small role in these conditions except as a means of facilitating the selection of vessels for duplex Doppler sampling.

Hepatic Tumors

Characteristic signal patterns from malignant tumors have been reported for continuous-wave, pulsed Doppler, and DCI.[36] The patterns that have been described generally involve the periphery of the tumor. With DCI these patterns include an increase in number of vessels and the presence of vessels of unusual course and caliber (Fig. 6-22).[5] Duplex ultrasound of these vessels typically reveals a Doppler spectrum with relatively high peak systolic velocities and a predominance of high power, low frequency components.[37] High-frequency (5 kHz or greater) shifts attributed to arterioportal shunting have been found in hepatomas and some metastatic tumors and appear relatively specific for highly vascular tumors.[38] In contrast to malignant tumors, which have high-velocity arteriovenous (AV) shunts, hemangiomas have slow flow and thus are not associated with abnormal Doppler signals (Fig. 6-23).

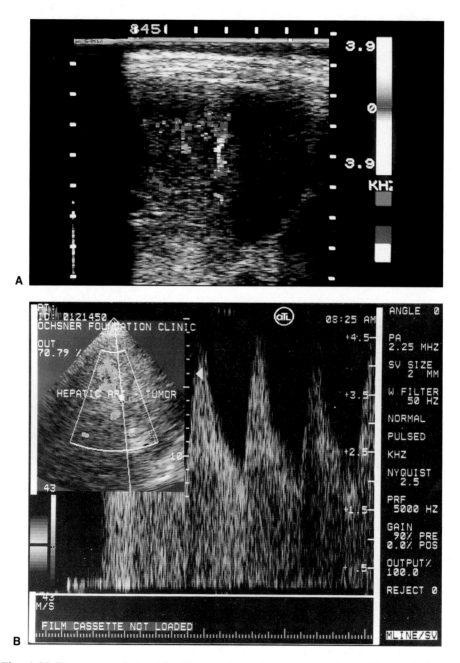

Fig. 6-22 Tumor vascularity. **(A)** Abnormal vessels are seen at the periphery of a hepatic metastasis from colon carcinoma. Spectral Doppler is required to confirm the abnormality. **(B)** Typical spectral changes associated with malignant vascularity are shown with high systolic and diastolic velocity and a low-impedance waveform.

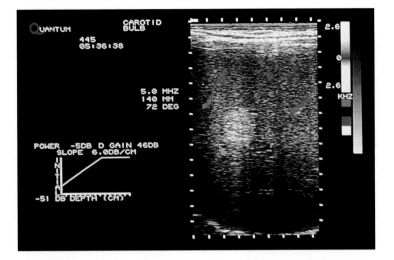

Fig. 6-23 Hemangioma. In contrast to the hypervascularity that may be seen with malignant tumors, hemangiomas have very slow flow and do not appear vascular on DCI.

SPLENIC AND MESENTERIC VESSELS

Examination of the splenic artery by DCI is possible but has little clinical utility. The origin of the splenic artery is from the celiac axis and may be identified in most patients. Similarly, the distal splenic artery at the level of the splenic hilum and its major branches into the spleen are visible by using the spleen as an acoustic window (Fig. 6-24). Splenic artery occlusion and aneurysms are potentially identifiable by DCI.

Detection of stenosis or occlusion of the superior mesenteric artery is potentially of greater clinical relevance, particularly in the work-up of patients with intestinal angina. In the past, diagnosis of mesenteric arterial occlusive disease has required arteriography, but a growing role for DCI and duplex Doppler sonography is likely (Fig. 6-25).

A major difficulty in the Doppler assessment of the splenic and mesenteric vessels is limited visualization resulting from superimposed intestinal gas. If the patient is thin and gas is minimal, the ability of DCI to image the splenic and mesenteric arteries and veins is excellent, permitting the diagnosis and characterization of stenosis and occlusion.

KIDNEYS

Doppler evaluation of the native kidney has, to date, proven to be of somewhat limited value because of inconsistent results. This is related to the location of the renal arteries, the common occurrence of multiple arteries, and the presence of superimposed bowel and bone. Although experience with DCI in the evaluation of the native kidney is limited, a combination of DCI and duplex Doppler measurements has the potential of increasing the utility of Doppler in the assessment of renal flow. DCI readily permits confirmation of arterial and venous patency in the kidney and is particularly useful when

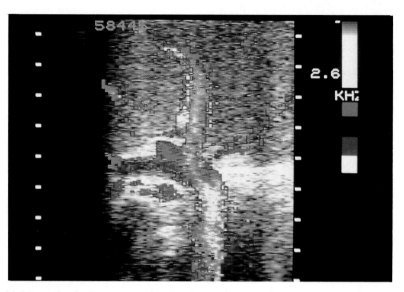

Fig. 6-24 Normal splenic artery and vein. Coronal image shows a patent splenic vein and its branches (blue) Segments of the splenic arteries within the spleen are also shown (red). (From Merritt,[5] with permission.)

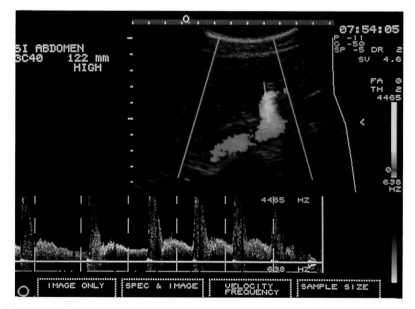

Fig. 6-25 Normal superior mesenteric artery. Longitudinal image shows the proximal portion of the SMA as it arises from the aorta. There is no evidence of narrowing or turbulence in the image. Spectral analysis shows a normal waveform for a fasting patient.

renal arterial occlusion or renal vein thrombosis is suspected. Interest in the use of Doppler as a screening method for renovascular hypertension is growing, and DCI should contribute to the development of more reliable methods for this purpose. In the evaluation of the transplanted kidney, DCI provides an extremely valuable adjunct to the imaging examination, allowing rapid identification of normal and abnormal arterial and venous flow.

Anatomy and Examination Technique

RENAL ARTERY AND VEIN

The renal arteries arise from the aorta at the level of the upper border of the second lumbar vertebra, approximately 1 cm caudal to the origin of the superior mesenteric artery (SMA). The SMA is therefore a useful landmark when beginning a search for the renal arteries. The renal arteries pass transversely across the crura of the diaphragm and upper portions of the psoas muscles to enter the kidneys. The right renal artery passes posterior to the IVC and is often visible in this location by ultrasound, particularly in parasagittal imaging planes. The level at which the right renal artery passes posterior to the IVC is usually within 1 or 2 cm of where the portal vein crosses anterior to the IVC, thus serving as a useful landmark. The right renal artery also passes posterior to the head of the pancreas and the second portion of the duodenum; if an anterior imaging approach is used, gas in the duodenum may hinder visualization of the vessel. The left renal artery lies posterior to the left renal vein and passes behind the pancreas and splenic vein. Accessory renal arteries are common, being reported in approximately 23 percent of the population. Accessory arteries are more common on the left side and tend to supply the inferior pole. In addition to arising from the aorta, accessory renal arteries may originate from the iliac and other abdominal vessels.[39] The high incidence of accessory renal arteries poses a significant problem in the sonographic assessment of renal artery stenosis. The renal veins both lie anterior to the arteries, with the right renal vein passing directly into the IVC. The left renal vein is longer than the right, passing anterior to the aorta and posterior to the pancreas, splenic vein, and SMA and superior mesenteric vein. With ultrasound, some dilatation of the left renal vein is commonly seen as a result of compression in the base of the mesentery as it passes between the aorta and the proximal SMA.

Within the kidney, the main renal arteries split into anterior and posterior segmental branches that then divide into a number of interlobar branches to supply apical, upper anterior, middle anterior, lower, and posterior segments of the kidney. Each of the five segments of the kidney is supplied by its own branch of the interlobar artery, and no collateral circulation exists between the segments. The relatively constant segmental distribution of the interlobar branches is important in the evaluation of intrarenal blood flow by DCI, because interruption of flow to individual segments of the kidney is possible with obstruction of these branches, and areas of segmental hypoperfusion may be identified by DCI. Within the kidneys, the interlobar vessels pass between the medullary columns and at the corticomedullary junction, giving rise to the arcuate arteries. From the arcuate arteries, small intralobular arteries arise and penetrate the cortex (Fig. 6-26)

Imaging of the main renal arteries in the native kidney is often possible, provided that a suitable acoustical window is found. Both supine and decubitus transabdominal as well as prone translumbar approaches may be helpful in visualizing the extrarenal segment of the renal arteries by DCI. Usually the renal arteries are imaged in the axial plane at the level of the SMA and the left renal vein (Fig. 6-27). In sagittal scan planes, identification

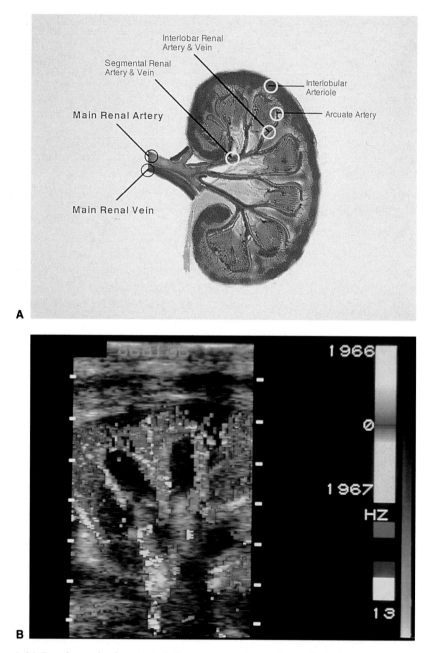

Fig. 6-26 Renal vessels (drawing). **(A)** Major vessels supplying the kidney. **(B)** DCI permits visualization of arcuate and interlobular branches too small to be recognized by gray-scale imaging.

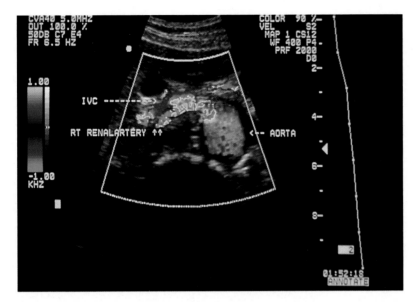

Fig. 6-27 Normal renal artery. Transverse image shows the proximal portion of the right renal artery as it passes behind the IVC. The mixture of colors in the renal artery does not indicate stenosis, but is largely a result of changes in the Doppler angle as the vessel passes to the right.

of the right renal artery as it passes posterior to the IVC may be helpful. The acoustical window provided by the liver and IVC makes evaluation of the right renal vessels easier to perform than on the left. In the presence of an enlarged spleen, access to the left kidney is improved. For examinations of adults, satisfactory penetration and flow sensitivity usually requires the use of 2.5- to 3.5-MHz transducers, with higher frequencies reserved for small patients and children.

With newer instruments, imaging of the segmental, interlobar, and, in some patients, arcuate arteries of the native kidneys is possible. These vessels are not visible by conventional duplex Doppler, and DCI aids in their localization for spectral sampling. The spectral waveform obtained from the main renal artery and its branches shows a pattern typical of a low-resistance vessel with high flow velocity persisting throughout diastole. DCI

is capable of showing the presence of flow throughout the cardiac cycle in the normal renal artery, provided that instrument settings (wall filter) have not been adjusted to limit the display of lower-frequency shifts present in diastole. Velocity measurements in the main renal artery are normally lower than 100 cm/s; however, values as high as 180 cm/s have been reported.[40] With DCI instruments, venous flow can be seen within the kidney as well as within the main renal veins and the identification of normal and symmetrical venous flow from the kidneys may be useful in excluding main renal vein thrombosis (Fig. 6-28).

Renal Artery Stenosis

Hypertension is a major medical problem, and renal artery stenosis is the single most common correctable cause of this condition.

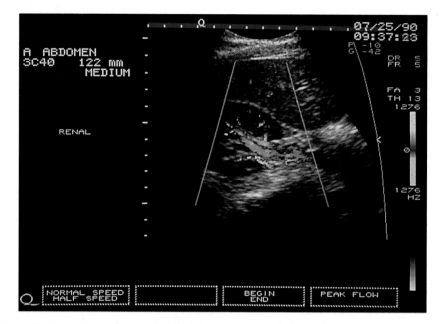

Fig. 6-28 Normal renal vein. Axial view of the right kidney shows a normal renal vein emerging from the renal hilus. DCI may aid in the identification of renal vein thrombosis and tumor invasion.

Thus, there is a great deal of interest in the use of noninvasive techniques for identification of significant renal artery stenosis in the hypertensive population. Duplex Doppler has shown varying degrees of success in permitting the diagnosis of renal artery stenosis and occlusion; the contributions of DCI to diagnosis have been recently investigated.[41,42] With duplex Doppler, the criteria for the diagnosis of significant (>50 percent) stenosis in the main renal artery have included the presence of systolic velocity greater than 100 cm/s,[43] a ratio of peak renal artery velocity to peak aortic velocity of 3.5 or greater,[44] spectral broadening, absence of diastolic flow, and lack of flow indicating occlusion. Using these criteria, sensitivities of 89 to 94 percent and specificities of 73 to 95 percent have been obtained in detecting significant stenosis.[40,43,44] Other investigators, using similar criteria, have reported much less encouraging results, noting a specificity for Doppler as poor as 37 percent.[42] Because

accurate evaluation demands that the entire course of each renal artery by examined, the study may be compromised in many patients as a result of superimposed bowel gas, bone, or fat. The accuracy of renal artery Doppler is impaired by difficulty in obtaining adequate samples from both renal arteries[45] and by the occurrence of multiple renal arteries in more than 20 percent of patients. With DCI, normal renal arteries and veins are regularly imaged in thin patients and children but are less consistently imaged in most adults. Criteria for diagnosis of stenosis by DCI include not only the spectral changes described with duplex Doppler but also the direct visualization of vessel narrowing and the stenotic jet. Despite the additional information that DCI is capable of providing, reports by Berland et al.[42] and Desberg et al.[41] do not show encouraging results. Berland et al. compared color duplex sonography with angiography in 26 patients. The major criterion for diagnosing a diameter narrowing of more than 50 percent was a velocity of greater than 100 cm/s. Accessory renal arteries were present in 22 percent of kidneys, but none of these were identified by DCI. Only 58 percent of the main arteries were identified by DCI. Angiography demonstrated 10 stenoses and one occlusion, but none of the stenotic vessels were identified by duplex scanning; the diagnosis of the single occluded vessel was correct. The specificity of ultrasound examination was only 37 percent. The study by Desberg et al.[41] evaluated 55 kidneys in 30 patients and compared the results of aortography and DCI. Doppler criteria for renal artery stenosis included a renal artery to aorta velocity ratio (RAR) of 3.5 greater and/or a renal artery peak systolic velocity (PSV) of greater than 100 cm/s. Doppler tracings were obtained in only 69 percent of 36 kidneys with a patent single renal artery, and both RAR and PSV results were insensitive in the diagnosis of renal artery stenosis. Accessory arteries were present in 24 percent of kidneys, but none were visualized by DCI. These findings led the authors to conclude that DCI is not an adequate screening method for the detection of renal artery stenosis.

In attempting to reconcile conflicting results reported in the literature regarding the efficacy of Doppler in providing clinically useful information in patients with renovascular hypertension, it is necessary to point out that these examinations require considerable skill and a meticulous and often time-consuming sampling of the renal artery. Careful attention to the audible changes in the Doppler signal, as well as to visible findings, is necessary. Since the vessel may not be visible even by DCI, hand–ear as well as hand–eye coordination to detect and record audible and visible Doppler changes is of particular importance. That the generally more positive results have come from vascular laboratories, where analysis of the audible Doppler signal receives emphasis, rather than from imaging departments may explain the differences re-

ported. With these thoughts in mind, it seems prudent, at least for the present, to be cautious in recommending the use of either duplex or color Doppler for initial screening of hypertensive patients for renal artery stenosis. The need for a simple, accurate, and noninvasive screening technique for renovascular disease will undoubtedly stimulate further interest in this application.

Renal Carcinoma

As in the liver, vascular changes associated with malignant tumors may be demonstrated by Doppler ultrasound.[4,46–48] With a Doppler frequency shift in excess of 2.5 kHz (for 3.0-MHz insonating frequency) as the criterion for diagnosis, tumor signals have been reported in up to 83 percent of untreated renal cell carcinomas, 75 percent of Wilms' tumors, as well as in metastases to the kidney, but not in association with benign renal masses.[46] Correlation with angiographic findings suggests that the high-frequency Doppler signals were associated with arteriovenous shunts. The sensitivity and specificity of Doppler in identifying malignant tumors of the kidney are reported to be 70 and 94 percent, respectively.[49] Doppler ultrasound adds useful information to the study of renal masses, and the detection of high-velocity signals can aid in the differential diagnosis of renal masses.[4] DCI has also been reported to show changes associated with renal carcinoma.[47] In our experience, increased vascularity is often seen in association with hypervascular renal carcinoma, and DCI aids in the selection of sampling sites to obtain the characteristic spectral abnormalities described above (Fig. 6-29). These methods are, however, limited in their ability to detect avascular tumors.

Other Renal Abnormalities

Renal obstruction has been shown to increase renal vascular resistance in animals, and there is evidence that this also occurs in humans.

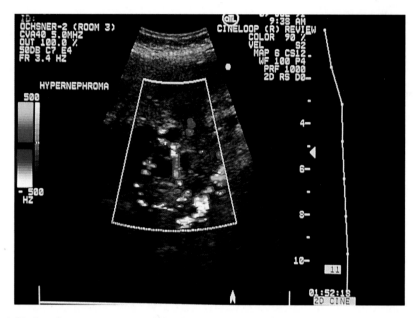

Fig. 6-29 Renal carcinoma. Image of hypervascular hypernephroma shows extensive tumor neovascularity. Spectral Doppler showed characteristic high-velocity low-impedance waveforms.

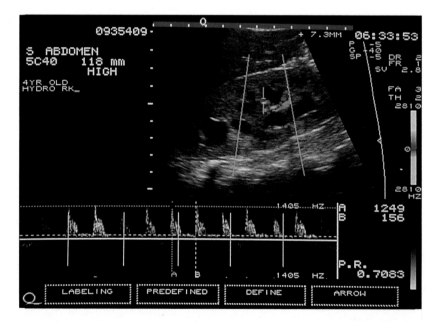

Fig. 6-30 Obstruction. Longitudinal view of the kidney of a 4-year-old child shows moderate hydronephrosis. DCI-guided Doppler sampling from an interlobar renal artery reveals an abnormal spectral waveform with reduced diastolic flow.

Duplex measurements of the RI show a significant difference between obstructed and nonobstructed kidneys. In normal kidneys, the RI measured in the interlobar arteries is usually less than 0.70.[50] When obstruction is present, higher values are encountered. An RI of 0.70 or greater appears to correlate well with obstruction, resulting in a sensitivity of 92 percent, a specificity of 88 percent, and an accuracy of 90 percent.[51] Doppler measurements are therefore quite promising in aiding the differentiation of obstructive from non-obstructive calycectasis. The use of DCI in this specific application has not been reported; however, the complementary nature of DCI and duplex sonography, using DCI to identify vessels for duplex sampling, is a strong recommendation for using DCI in this examination (Fig. 6-30).

Experience with Doppler ultrasonography in renal vein thrombosis is limited, but our experience with DCI in patients in whom size and gas do not prevent assessment is encouraging. The demonstration of a distended renal vein without evidence of flow has correlated well with other studies in indicating renal vein thrombosis in a small number of patients. DCI is also useful in confirming tumor invasion of the renal veins when imaging findings are equivocal. With DCI, intrarenal vessels including segmental, interlobar, and arcuate vessels are visible in many patients, and we have noted diminished patterns of flow in these vessels in patients with advanced renal parenchymal disease. The future role of DCI in the evaluation of renal perfusion remains to be defined, but the capabilities provided by new imaging methods are promising and deserve further study.

Renal Transplantation

Transplant dysfunction may result from vessel stenosis, occlusion, or parenchymal changes secondary to rejection, tubular necrosis, or drug toxicity. The ability of Doppler ultrasonography to assess major vessels

for primary abnormalities, as well as documentation of dynamics of flow that reflect changes in smaller vessels, has encouraged routine postoperative use of ultrasound in the evaluation of renal transplants. Because of the superficial location of the transplanted kidney and the lack of superimposed gas, high-quality duplex and DCI studies are possible in essentially all patients. DCI can be performed at 5.0 to 7.5 MHz, permitting excellent detail of intrarenal and extrarenal vessels (Fig. 6-31). DCI examinations permit rapid and accurate diagnosis of stenosis or thrombosis of the main renal artery and vein, and we believe that DCI is the procedure of choice for the initial evaluation of the main renal vessels for patency or significant stenosis (Fig. 6-32). Evidence supporting the role of DCI in detecting intra- or extrarenal vascular complications of renal transplants has been provided by Grenier et al.[52] in a study of 146 renal allografts. In this study, DCI correctly identified 30 of 34 vascular complications, including 10 of 11 significant stenoses of the renal artery or one of its main branches. There were two false-positive diagnoses of renal artery stenoses. Nine of nine renal artery thromboses and the single pseudoaneurysm were also identified. DCI also demonstrated five of five segmental infarcts, two of two postbiopsy arteriovenous fistulas, and three of six segmental or interlobar artery stenoses.

In the normal transplant, flow in the segmental, interlobar, and arcuate vessels continues throughout both systole and diastole, and RI values range from 0.50 to 0.70 in the segmental and interlobar arteries. When duplex Doppler was used, significant differences in perfusion patterns from normal have been observed, with elevation of RI values in patients with rejection and acute tubular necrosis.[53] DCI provides a clue to some of the more severe changes in renal perfusion by displaying alterations of the duration of arterial flow in systole, with the duration of the display of systolic flow decreasing as the

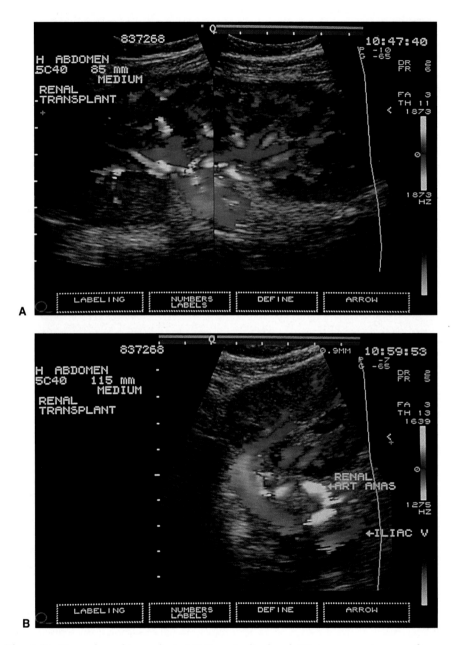

Fig. 6-31 Normal renal transplant. **(A)** Longitudinal and **(B)** transverse images of a normal renal transplant show the ability of DCI to provide detailed information of renal arterial and venous flow. In Figure A the segmental, interlobar, arcuate, and interlobular branches are seen. In Fig. B the main renal artery and vein and anastomoses to the iliac vessels are shown.

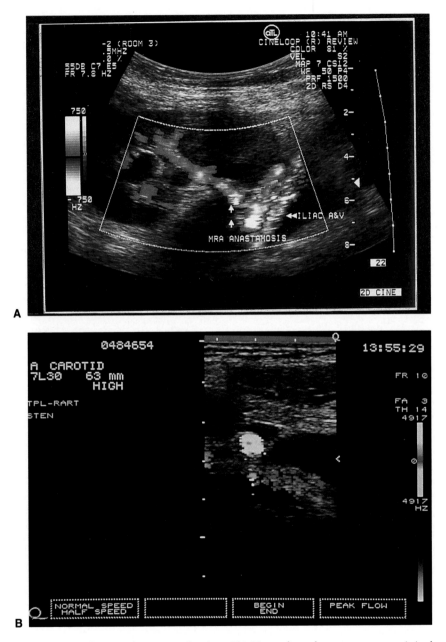

Fig. 6-32 Transplant renal artery evaluation. **(A)** Normal renal artery anastomosis is shown. **(B)** DCI of transplanted renal artery near the anastomosis reveals a mosaic pattern of colors associated with a bruit. (*Figure continues.*)

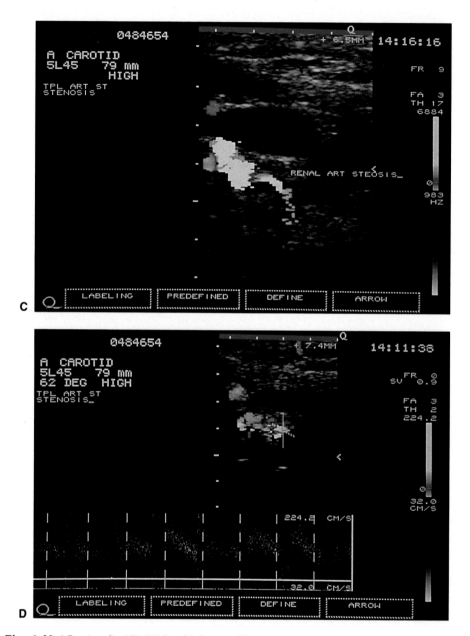

Fig. 6-32 (*Continued*). **(C)** With a high-pass filter to suppress the signal from the bruit, a high-velocity jet is seen at the anastomosis of the main renal artery and the iliac artery. **(D)** Spectral Doppler confirms stenosis with velocities exceeding 225 cm/s. (*Figure continues.*)

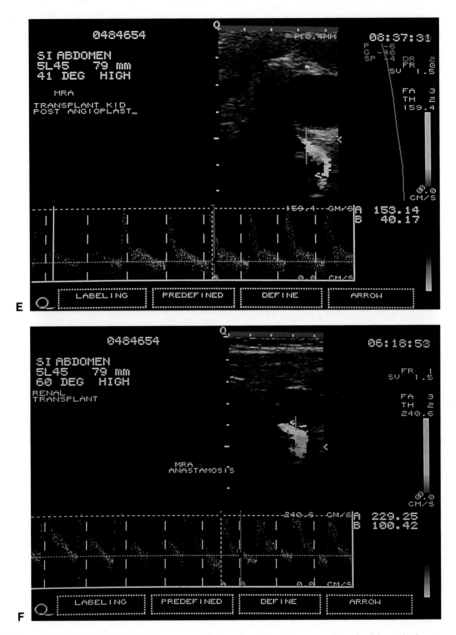

Fig. 6-32 (*Continued*). **(E)** After angioplasty, the velocities are reduced, although the stenosis has not been completely eliminated. **(F)** A follow-up study shows restenosis with velocities again in excess of 225 cm/s.

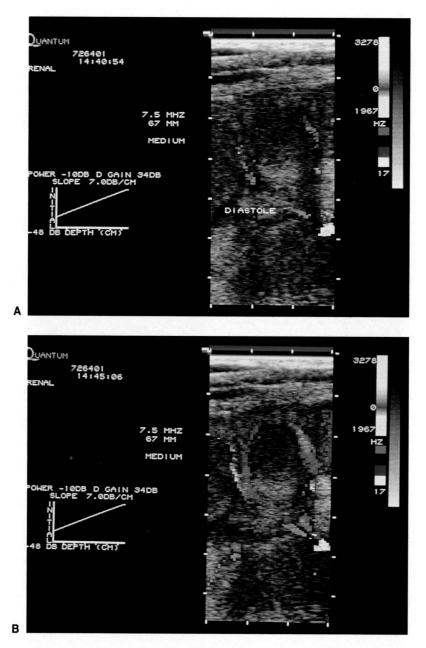

Fig. 6-33 Transplant rejection. Although DCI does not replace pulsed-Doppler analysis of renal artery flow, gross changes in renal perfusion may be seen by DCI. **(A)** In systole, flow is seen in interlobar arteries and veins. **(B)** In diastole, arterial flow is not seen. In a normal transplant, arterial flow continues throughout diastole. In this patient with rejection, the DCI pattern indicates an increase in the RI. (From Merritt,[20] with permission.)

RI in the renal artery increases (Fig. 6-33). Nishioka et al.[54] have correlated the visualization of segmental and parenchymal branches of the renal artery by using DCI with transplant function. Vessel visualization was correlated with impaired graft function. Changes were more pronounced in the parenchymal vessel. Although these authors considered the visibility of renal vessels by DCI to be useful, they did not suggest replacing quantitative measurement of flow parameters with Doppler spectral analysis. The ability of DCI to provide an overall view of transplant perfusion was, however, found to be valuable, and clinical use of the analysis of flow imaging patterns was recommended. A comparison of DCI and duplex Doppler in the evaluation of 50 renal allografts performed by Mostbeck et al.[55] has revealed a good correlation of measurements of RIs and DCI findings. All five allografts with pathologic RI measurements greater than or equal to 0.9 showed abnormal color flow characterized by absence of flow in arcuate and/or interlobar arteries, leading the authors to conclude that a normal color flow pattern excludes severe vascular compromise to the allograft. In addition, DCI revealed three biopsy-related vascular lesions, two of which had been missed by duplex Doppler.

Our experience confirms the value of the subjective overall assessment of renal transplant blood flow provided by DCI, and we believe that DCI is an extremely useful adjunct to analysis of the Doppler spectrum. As in other organs, the ability to visualize small vessels within the kidney aids in the selection of sampling sites for spectral Doppler.

Although high RIs have been associated with acute rejection, other causes of RI elevation including acute tubular necrosis, renal vein thrombosis, renal compression, pyelonephritis, and obstruction have been described

and lack of RI elevation in patients with acute transplant rejection has also been reported.[56-61] The importance of correlation of Doppler spectral analysis, imaging, and clinical observations in determining the most likely cause of transplant dysfunction deserves emphasis.[62]

A particularly useful application of DCI is in the identification of complications following biopsy of renal transplants. The ability of DCI to provide a global view of normal and disturbed flow makes it an especially powerful tool in this application. Routine evaluation of kidneys with DCI following transplant biopsy commonly reveals small AV fistulas that are not clinically apparent. We have monitored a small number of these lesions and found that at least some regress spontaneously. At least two studies have confirmed the value of DCI in identification of postbiopsy complications. DCI findings in eight patients with postbiopsy renal transplant AV fistulas have been reported by Middleton et al.[63] Localized tissue vibration, appearing as random color assignment in extravascular renal parenchyma adjacent to the fistula, was seen in six of the eight patients (Fig. 6-34). Confirmation of the AV fistula was provided by spectral analysis, which revealed decreased RIs of 0.31 to 0.50 in all eight patients and increased flow velocities in seven of the eight patients. Arterialization of the venous waveform from the draining vein was also documented in all patients. In six patients, the increased flow velocities resulted in increased color saturation toward white in the supplying artery or draining vein. DCI is superior to duplex ultrasound in identification of AV fistulas and pseudoaneurysms; therefore, DCI is recommended as the method of choice for noninvasive detection of vascular lesions due to percutaneous biopsy. A study of 100 patients with renal allografts 1 to 30 days following biopsy has been reported by Hübsch et al.[64] In six

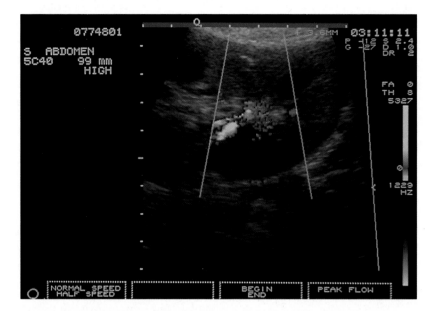

Fig. 6-34 Renal arteriovenous fistula. A mosaic pattern of color resulting from tissue vibration associated with a bruit is seen in the kidney following renal biopsy. The changes are the result of a small AV fistula caused by the biopsy. The abnormality resolved spontaneously. The DCI pattern associated with a bruit is an extremely important clue to the presence of subtle vascular abnormalities including AV fistulas and stenoses.

patients DCI demonstrated areas of disturbed flow confirmed by intra-arterial digital subtraction angiography to be related to AV fistulas in four patients and pseudoaneurysms in two. These findings led the authors to conclude that DCI is the method of choice for noninvasive detection of vascular lesions due to percutaneous biopsy.

OTHER ABDOMINAL APPLICATIONS

Aorta and Inferior Vena Cava

Conventional real-time gray-scale imaging is useful in the diagnosis and follow-up of abdominal aortic aneurysms, and DCI adds little if any information. Often the visibility of the iliac arteries is improved by the use of

DCI, and extension of aneurysms of the aortic bifurcation into the iliac arteries can be better documented by DCI than by conventional imaging alone. The ability of DCI to image flow aids in the identification of hypoechoic thrombus within an aneurysm and also demonstrates turbulent flow patterns. This information is, however, of little clinical value. In dissection of the aorta, DCI is more useful. DCI provides confirmation of dissection and aids in differentiating the true lumen from the false lumen (Fig. 6-35). In our experience, flow in the false lumen frequently is in the same direction as in the true lumen only briefly during early systole. In the false lumen, flow reverses in late systole and diastole. Presumably this is due to increased resistance in the false lumen and pressure gradients between the true and false channels.

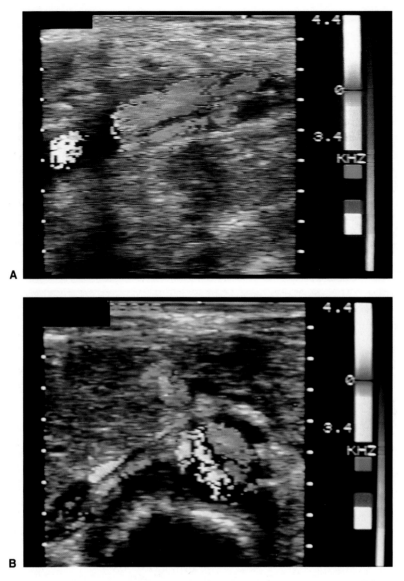

Fig. 6-35 Aortic dissection. **(A)** Longitudinal and **(B)** transverse images of dissecting aneurysm of the abdominal aorta. The true lumen is anterior, and the false lumen is posterior. The right renal artery is seen to arise from the false lumen in the transverse image.

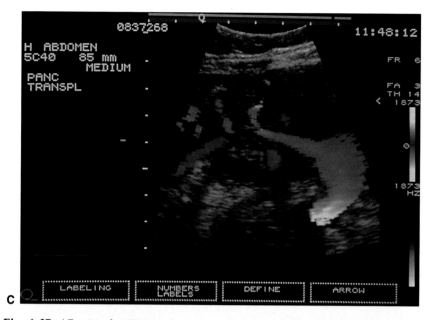

Fig. 6-37 *(Continued)*. **(C)** Portal vein anastomosis of pancreatic transplant is shown.

DCI aids in the evaluation of the IVC when thrombosis or tumor invasion is suspected (Fig. 6-36). Partial occlusion may be differentiated from complete occlusion with greater confidence than by conventional ultrasound imaging alone, and collateral vessels not seen by conventional imaging may be detected.

Pancreatic Transplantation

As in renal and hepatic transplants, the integrity of the arterial and venous supply is critical in pancreatic transplantation. The transplanted pancreas, like the kidney, is superficial and is therefore well suited to examination by ultrasound. The arterial supply of the pancreatic allograft is from the celiac artery and the SMA. These vessels are anastomosed to the iliac artery. The portal vein is anastomosed to the external iliac vein to provide venous drainage, and pancreatic secretions are drained by duodenocystostomy. Graft ischemia is an important cause of transplant failure in the early post-transplant period, and duplex Doppler is commonly used to monitor postoperative blood flow to the pancreas.[65,66] We have found DCI to be a valuable adjunct to duplex Doppler sonography in the assessment of blood flow to the transplanted pancreas, permitting early identification of mechanical problems with arterial and venous anastomoses (Fig. 6-37). The iliac artery and vein are examined to identify the anastomoses of the celiac artery, the SMA, and the portal vein. Flow within the body of the pancreas is easily confirmed by visualization of the splenic artery and vein along the posterior aspect of the allograft.

Detection of Tumor Neovascularity

The use of DCI to detect tumor vascularity in the liver and kidneys has been noted earlier in this chapter. Doppler has also been used in the evaluation of tumors elsewhere in the abdomen.[67] With duplex methods, high sensitivity is required to detect the low-amplitude signals present in tumor vessels, and careful Doppler investigation of the margin of the tumor is required to identify the vessels

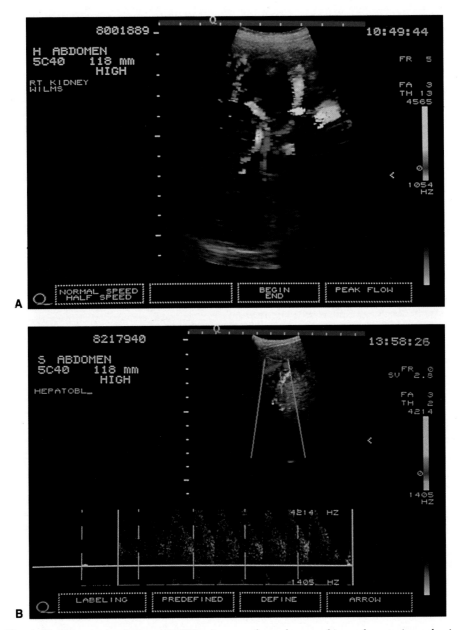

Fig. 6-38 Tumor vascularity. **(A)** Wilms' tumor shows large and irregular arteries and veins. **(B)** Hepatoblastoma likewise shows a focal increase in vessels near a tumor nodule within the liver. Unlike normal hepatic vessels, tumor neovascularity is characterized by an increase in the size and number of vessels, often with irregular caliber and course. Pulsed Doppler shows elevated velocity and low impedance.

of interest. As noted previously, DCI has the potential of aiding the evaluation of tumor vascularity by providing visual identification of abnormal vessels for spectral Doppler sampling (Fig. 6-38). The use of DCI with ultasound contrast agents may, in the future, further enhance the role of ultrasonography in tumor analysis.[68]

SUMMARY

Abdominal applications of Doppler ultrasonography are becoming increasingly important as familiarity with Doppler principles and instruments grows. The availability of sensitive duplex and DCI instruments specifically adapted for use in the abdomen and pelvis has stimulated interest in the use of Doppler techniques as a complement to conventional imaging. Although the simultaneous display of tissue and flow information has enhanced the ease of evaluation of vascular abnormalities and increased diagnostic confidence, the role of Doppler is only just beginning to be defined. Since blood flow is a fundamental factor in health and disease, it is hoped that the new information provided by Doppler evaluation of the abdomen will continue to advance the role of ultrasound as a primary diagnostic method as Doppler and color imaging technology mature.

ACKNOWLEDGMENTS

This chapter reflects in large part the dedicated work of the sonography staff of the Alton Ochsner Medical Institutions. Special thanks are due to the sonographers who have participated with energy and enthusiasm in our involvement with DCI over the past 6 years: Steve Bernhardt, RDMS; Lauren Althans, RDMS; Laurie Troxclair, RDMS; Lisa Schuler, RDMS; Michele Bienvenu, RDMS; and William Perret, RDMS. Appreciation is also expressed to Benita Berthel, RDMS, and her students in the School of Ultrasonography of the Alton Ochsner Medical Institutions.

REFERENCES

1. Merritt CRB: Editorial. Ultrasound safety—what are the issues. Radiology 173:304, 1989
2. Taylor KJW, Burns PN: Duplex Doppler scanning in the pelvis and abdomen. Ultrasound Med Biol 11:643, 1985
3. Wells PNT, Halliwell M, Skidmore R, et al: Tumour detection by ultrasonic Doppler blood-flow signals. Ultrasonics 15:231, 1977
4. Dubbins PA, Wells I: Renal carcinoma: duplex Doppler evaluation. Br J Radiol 59:231, 1986
5. Merritt CRB: Doppler color flow imaging. J Clin Ultrasound 15:591, 1987
6. Merritt CRB: Ultrasonographic demonstration of portal vein thrombosis. Radiology, 133:425, 1979
7. Van Gansbeke D, Avni EF, Delcour C, et al: Sonographic features of portal vein thrombosis. AJR 144:749, 1985
8. Merritt CRB: Ultrasonographic evaluation of the retrocaval region. Crit Rev Diagn Imaging 20:215, 1983
9. Merritt CRB, Goldsmith JP, Sharp MJ: Sonographic detection of portal venous gas in infants with necrotizing enterocolitis. AJR 143:1059, 1984
10. Sexton CC, Zeman RK: Correlation of computed tomography, sonography, and gross anatomy of the liver. AJR 141:711, 1983
11. Hosoki T, Kuroda C, Tokunaga K, et al: Hepatic venous outflow obstruction: evaluation with pulsed duplex sonography. Radiology 170:733, 1989
12. Ohnishi K, Terabayashi H, Tsunoda T, Nomura F: Budd-Chiari syndrome: diagnosis with duplex sonography. Am J Gastroenterol 85:165, 1990
13. Grant EG, Perrella R, Tessler FN, et al: Budd-Chiari syndrome: the results of duplex and color Doppler imaging. AJR 152:377, 1989
14. Vogelzang RL, Anschuetz SL, Gore RM: Budd-Chiari syndrome: CT observations. Radiology 163:329, 1987
15. Grant EG, Tessler FN, Gomes AS et al: Color Doppler imaging of portosystemic shunts. AJR 154:393, 1990
16. Dawson JL: Normal anatomy. p. 7. In Wright R, Alberti KGGM, Karran S, Millward-Sadler GH (eds): Liver and Biliary Disease. WB Saunders, Philadelphia, 1979
17. Atri M, de Stempel J, Bret PM, Illescas FF:

Incidence of portal vein thrombosis complicating liver metastasis as detected by duplex ultrasound. J Ultrasound Med 9:285, 1990

18. Valla D, Casadevall N, Huisse MG, et al: Etiology of portal vein thrombosis in adults. A prospective evaluation of primary myeloproliferative disorders. Gastroenterology 9:1063, 1988

19. Slovis TL, Haller JO, Cohen HL, et al: Complicated appendiceal inflammatory disease in children: pylephlebitis and liver abscess. Radiology 171:823, 1989

20. Merritt CRB: Real-time Doppler color-flow imaging: other applications. p. 42. In Bernstein EF (ed): Recent Advances in Noninvasive Diagnostic Techniques in Vascular Disease. CV Mosby, St. Louis, 1990

21. Miller VE, Berland LL: Pulsed Doppler duplex sonography and CT of portal vein thrombosis. AJR 145:73, 1985

22. Alpern MB, Rubin JM, Williams DM, Capek D: Porta hepatis: duplex Doppler US with angiographic correlation. Radiology 162:53, 1987

23. Ralls PW, Lee KP, Mayekawa DS, et al: Color Doppler sonography of portocaval shunts. J Clin Ultrasound 18:379, 1990

24. Bezzi M, Mitchell DG, Needleman L, Goldberg BB: Iatrogenic aneurysmal portal-hepatic venous fistula. Diagnosis by color Doppler imaging. J Ultrasound Med 7:457, 1988

25. Ralls PW, Quinn MF, Rogers W, Halls J: Sonographic anatomy of the hepatic artery. AJR 136:1059, 1981

26. Berland LL, Lawson TL, Foley WD: Porta hepatis: sonographic discrimination of bile ducts from arteries with pulsed Doppler with new anatomic criteria. AJR 138:833, 1982

27. Ralls PW: Color Doppler sonography of the hepatic artery and portal venous system. AJR 155:517, 1990

28. Bret PM, Reinhold C, Herba M, et al: Replaced or right accessory hepatic artery: can ultrasound replace angiography? J Clin Ultrasound 16:245, 1988

29. Merritt CRB: Vascular accidents: aneurysms and thrombosis of the hepatic, splenic, and portal vessels. p. 198. In Serafini AN, Guter M (eds): Medical Imaging of the Liver and Spleen. Appleton-Century-Crofts, East Norwalk, CT, 1983

30. Endress C, Kling GA, Medrazo BL: Diagnosis of hepatic artery aneurysm with portal vein fistula using image-directed Doppler ultrasound. J Clin Ultrasound 17:206, 1989

31. Segel MC, Zajko AB, Bowen A, et al: Hepatic artery thrombosis after liver transplantation: radiologic evaluation. AJR 146:137, 1986

32. Flint EW, Sumkin JH, Zajko AB, Bowen A: Duplex sonography of hepatic artery thrombosis after liver transplantation. AJR 151:481, 1988

33. Hidalgo EG, Abad J, Cantarero JM, et al: High-dose intra-arterial urokinase for the treatment of hepatic artery thrombosis in liver transplantation. Hepatogastroenterology 36:529, 1989

34. Zonderland HM, Lameris JS, Terpstra OT, et al: Auxiliary partial liver transplantation: imaging evaluation in 10 patients. AJR 153:981, 1989

35. Taylor KJ, Morse SS, Weltin GG, et al: Liver transplant recipients: portable duplex US with correlative angiography. Radiology 159:357, 1986

36. Taylor KJW, Ramos I, Carter D, et al: Correlation of Doppler US tumor signals with neovascular morphologic features. Radiology 166:57, 1988

37. Taylor KJ, Ramos I, Morse SS, et al: Focal liver masses: differential diagnosis with pulsed Doppler US. Radiology 164:643, 1987

38. Scoutt LM, Zawin ML, Taylor KJE: Doppler US. Part II. Clinical applications. Radiology 174:309, 1990

39. Woodburne RT: Essentials of Human Anatomy. Oxford University Press, New York, 1961

40. Hoffman U, Carter S, Goldman ML, et al: The role of duplex scanning for the detection of atherosclerotic renal artery disease. (in press)

41. Desberg AL, Paushter DM, Lammert GK, et al: Renal artery stenosis: evaluation with color Doppler flow imaging. Radiology 177:749, 1990

42. Berland LL, Koslin DB, Routh WD, Keller FS: Renal artery stenosis: prospective evaluation of diagnosis with color duplex US compared with angiography. Work in progress. Radiology 174:421, 1990

43. Avasthi PS, Voyles WF, Greene ER: Noninvasive diagnosis of renal artery stenosis by echo-Doppler velocimetry. Kidney Int 25:824, 1984

44. Kohler TR, Zierler RE, Martin RL, et al:

Noninvasive diagnosis of renal artery stenosis by ultrasonic duplex scanning. J Vasc Surg 4:450, 1986

45. Dubbins PA: Renal artery stenosis: duplex Doppler evaluation. Br J Radiol 59:225, 1986

46. Ramos IM, Taylor KJW, Kier R, et al: Tumor vascular signals in renal masses: detection with Doppler US. Radiology 168:633, 1988

47. Shimamoto K, Sakuma S, Ishigaki T, Makino N: Intratumoral blood flow: evaluation with color Doppler echography. Radiology 165:683, 1987

48. Kuijpers D, Jaspers R: Renal masses: differential diagnosis with pulsed Doppler US. Radiology 170:59, 1989

49. Kier R, Taylor KJW, Feyock AL, Ramos IM: Renal masses: characterization with Doppler US. Radiology 176:703, 1990

50. Gottlieb RH, Luhmann K IV, Oates RP: Duplex ultrasound evaluation of normal native kidneys and native kidneys with urinary tract obstruction. J Ultrasound Med 8:609, 1989

51. Platt JF, Rubin JM, Ellis JH: Distinction between obstructive and nonobstructive pyelocaliectasis with duplex Doppler sonography. AJR 153:997, 1989

52. Grenier N, Douws C, Morel D, et al: Detection of vascular complications in renal allografts with color Doppler flow imaging. Radiology 178:217, 1991

53. Rigsby CM, Taylor KJW, Weltin GG, et al: Renal allografts in acute rejection: evaluation using duplex sonography. Radiology 158:375, 1986

54. Nishioka N, Ikegami M, Imanishi M, et al: Renal transplant blood flow evaluation by color Doppler echography. Transplant Proc 21:1919, 1989

55. Mostbeck GH, Reichhalter C, Stockenhuber F, et al: Comparison of duplex sonography and color Doppler imaging in renal allograft evaluation: a prospective study. Eur J Radiol 10:201, 1990

56. Rifkin MD, Needleman L, Pasto ME, et al: Evaluation of renal transplant rejection by duplex Doppler examination: value of the resistive index. AJR 148:759, 1987

57. Buckley AR, Cooperberg PL, Reeve CE, Magil AB: The distinction between acute renal transplant rejection and cyclosporine nephrotoxicity: value of duplex sonography. AJR 149:521, 1987

58. Warshauer DM, Taylor KJW, Bia MJ, et al: Unusual causes of increased vascular impedance in renal transplants: duplex Doppler evaluation. Radiology 169:367, 1988

59. Allen KS, Jorkasky DK, Arger PH, et al: Renal allografts: prospective analysis of Doppler sonography. Radiology 169:371, 1988

60. Genkins SM, Sanfilippo FP, Carroll BA: Duplex Doppler sonography of renal transplants: lack of sensitivity and specificity in establishing pathologic diagnosis. AJR 152:535, 1989

61. Kelcz F, Pozniak MA, Pirsch JD, Oberly TD: Pyramidal appearance and resistive index: insensitive and nonspecific sonographic indicators of renal transplant rejection. AJR 155:531, 1990

62. Taylor KJW, Marks WH: Use of Doppler imaging for evaluation of dysfunction in renal allografts. Commentary. AJR 155:536, 1990

63. Middleton WD, Kellman GM, Melson GL, Madrazo BL: Postbiopsy renal transplant arteriovenous fistulas: color Doppler US characteristics. Radiology 171:253, 1989

64. Hübsch PJ, Mostbeck G, Barton PP, et al: Evaluation of arteriovenous fistulas and pseudoaneurysms in renal allografts following percutaneous needle biopsy. Color-coded Doppler sonography versus duplex Doppler sonography. Ultrasound Med 9:95, 1990

65. Boiskin I, Sandler MP, Fleischer AC, Nylander WA: Acute venous thrombosis after pancreas transplantation: diagnosis with duplex Doppler sonography and scintigraphy. AJR 154:529, 1990

66. Patel B, Wolverson MK, Mahanta B: Pancreatic transplant rejection: assessment with duplex US. Radiology 173:131, 1989

67. Orr NM, Taylor KJW: Doppler detection of tumor vascularity. p. 149. In Taylor KJW, Strandness DE (eds): Duplex Doppler Ultrasound. Churchill Livingstone, New York, 1990

68. Goldberg BB, Hilpert PL, Burns PN, et al: Hepatic tumors: signal enhancement at Doppler US after intravenous injection of a contrast agent. Radiology 177:713, 1990

7

Obstetric and Gynecologic Applications

Kenneth J. W. Taylor
Christopher R. B. Merritt
Lynwood Hammers
John S. Pellerito
Cara Case

The recent introduction of endovaginal Doppler color imaging (DCI) has produced a remarkable change in the diagnostic potential for pelvic ultrasound. The close proximity of the imaging probe to the target organs, the use of higher frequencies, and the absence of subcutaneous fat with its resultant artifact have dramatically improved the quality of ultrasound images, especially in obese patients, in whom clinical evaluation and transabdominal ultrasound had hitherto been most limited. The subsequent addition of pulsed Doppler has added much new information about the physiologic variations and flow in the uterine vessels during pregnancy and in the ovaries during the menstrual cycle. The addition of color Doppler yields a vas-cular map similar to a color anatomic illustration and expedites the location of vessels for pulsed-Doppler interrogation. The diagnostic capabilities of these techniques have yet to be fully defined. However, it is already apparent that these techniques can help in the differential diagnosis of many complications in the first trimester of pregnancy and can yield much data on both physiologic and pathologic conditions in the female pelvis.

NORMAL ANATOMY

Examination techniques for endovaginal ultrasonography (EVUS) by DCI are similar to those used for non-Doppler examinations

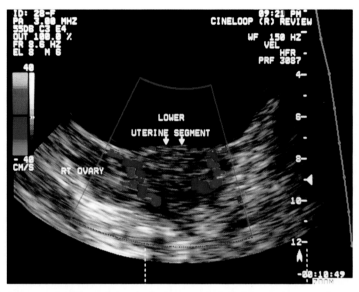

Fig. 7-3 Pelvic vessels. Transabdominal ultrasound showing uterine vessels on either side of the uterus and the arcuate branches.

In the region of the cervix, the main uterine arteries will be seen as they cross the floor of the pelvis and approach the cervix (Fig. 7-4). During examination of the uterus, small arcuate branches may be seen spreading horizontally from the main uterine vessels. Spectral analysis of the pulsed-Doppler waveform from the uterine arteries of a nonpregnant patient shows a normal pattern of relatively high-impedance flow (Fig. 7-4).

The examination is continued by angling the transducer toward one of the adnexa. The ovary should first be located. The diagnostic feature of the ovary, at least during reproductive years, is the presence of one or more follicles (Fig. 7-5A). The ovarian artery may be seen entering the ovary; if it is seen it usually shows a high-impedance flow pattern.

Blood flow within the ovary is affected by the menstrual cycle and pregnancy. Arteries within the nonfunctioning ovary show a high-impedance flow pattern (Fig. 7-5B). Low-impedance flow, seen in the luteal phase within the ovary, appears as a small glowing area perhaps 1 cm in diameter, either red or blue depending on the direction of flow (Fig. 7-5C). Luteal cysts are common and may show color and low-impedance flow around the periphery of the cyst. This low-impedance flow is first noticed around day 8 of the cycle and becomes more obvious between ovulation and approximately day 21, during the function of the corpus luteum (Fig. 7-5D). This luteal flow is also easily seen in the first trimester of all pregnancies. The most likely cause of these luteal flow patterns is neovascularization around the corpus luteum (Fig. 7-6).

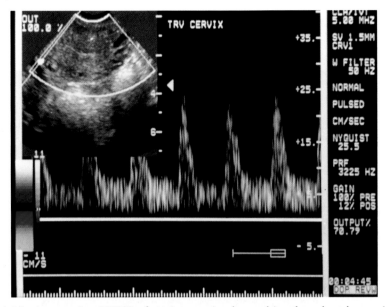

Fig. 7-4 Uterine arteries. EVUS of uterine arteries detected just lateral to the cervix. Note the continual diastolic flow but with a high impedance pattern (patient was 3 days post-therapeutic abortion).

The iliac vessels are seen most commonly immediately below the ovary. The largest vessel with the most obvious flow is the iliac vein (Fig. 7-7A). Pulsed-Doppler examination of this vessel demonstrates either continuous flow toward the heart or flow showing respiratory variation. Fusion of the external and internal iliac veins with the common iliac veins may be seen (Fig. 7-7B).

The external iliac artery is seen immediately adjacent to the vein, with flash filling seen only during systole. During diastole, reverse flow produces a blue coloration caused by the rebound of blood from the high impedance due to vasoconstriction in the muscle arterioles of the leg at rest (Fig. 7-8A).

By contrast, the internal iliac artery shows continuous forward flow in diastole (Fig. 7-8B). The remainder of the examination varies with the transducer design. With end-fire transducers, the maneuvers described will have demonstrated the cul-de-sac adequately. However, with the 30-degree offset transducer angled anteriorly, it is necessary to rotate the transducer through a full 360 degrees to ensure visualization of the cul-de-sac.

BIOEFFECTS CONSIDERATIONS

The complete safety of ultrasound in early pregnancy has not been entirely established. The argument for the safety of ultrasound most frequently made is that it has been used

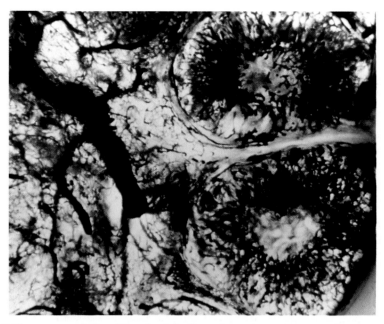

Fig. 7-6 Tumor vascularity. Vascular injection of rat ovary demonstrating two well-developed corpora lutea with surrounding neovascularization.

for two decades without any evidence of ill effects, at least in the few epidemiologic studies that have been reported.[1] However, caution is still appropriate for several reasons. First, ultrasound, and particularly EVUS, is now being used on an unprecedented scale earlier in pregnancy, and just before conception (during follicular monitoring). Second, the endovaginal route implies less attenuation of the ultrasound beam before it insonates the fetus or ovaries. Finally, the use of pulsed Doppler may involve the use of a considerably higher intensity than that used for imaging. In the second and third trimesters, the presence of fetal bone in the Doppler sample volume may result in conditions in which some localized heating of tissues may occur if high acoustic power is applied for an extended period. For these reasons, it is prudent to use the lowest intensity of ultrasound consistent with obtaining the required clinical data and to minimize the time of exposure.[2]

Clearly, for applications summarized in this chapter, pulsed and color Doppler are essential for evaluation of some of the complications of pregnancy. It is incumbent on the physicians who use it, however, to know the output of the Doppler device, to minimize both the intensity and time of exposure, and to use it only when the clinical benefit is likely to overwhelm the potential for harm, in keeping with the concept of ALARA (as low as reasonably achievable) discussed in Chapter 2 (p. 54). For example, ectopic pregnancy is a potentially lethal condition, and when it is suspected the transient use of Doppler is well justified if it can clarify the diagnosis. By contrast, we do not insonate a normal intrauterine sac but instead use Doppler to differentiate between an abnormal sac and a pseudosac, as will be described. Thus, we believe that Doppler ultrasound can be used prudently in pregnancy without producing any hazard to the developing fetus.

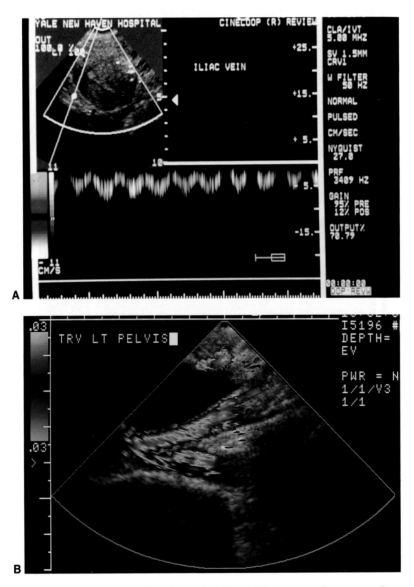

Fig. 7-7 Iliac veins. **(A)** EVUS showing color flow of iliac vein and corresponding pulsed–Doppler spectrum with the typical physiologic variations. **(B)** Color Doppler showing fusion of internal and external iliac veins into the common iliac vein.

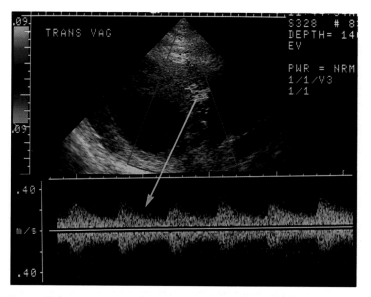

Fig. 7-10 Placental flow. Montage of pulsed and color EVUS showing well-developed placental flow by DCI and typical low-impedance flow by pulsed Doppler (arrow).

the placental vascularity and minimizes exposure of products of conception to ultrasonic energy.

SECOND AND THIRD TRIMESTERS OF PREGNANCY

In the second and third trimesters of pregnancy, the primary use of Doppler ultrasound has been in the assessment of flow in the umbilical and uterine arteries and, to a lesser extent, in the fetal aorta and carotid arteries. Using pulsed Doppler, most studies have investigated the relationship of changes in the fetal and uteroplacental circulation to conditions associated with intrauterine growth retardation, maternal hypertension, fetal anemias, and congenital anomalies.[8–10] DCI now provides a valuable adjunct to real-time imaging of the fetus in the second and third trimesters and aids in pulsed-Doppler examination. With DCI, the structural in-

formation provided by the real-time ultrasound image can be combined with the graphic display of fetal, placental, and uterine vasculature, aiding in the determination of normal development and function.

Pulsed-Doppler Guidance

A particularly important use of DCI is in the selection of optimal sites for pulsed-Doppler sampling within the fetus (Figs. 7-11 to 7-13). The selection of a sampling site for umbilical arterial Doppler sampling has been shown to have a significant influence on the accuracy of measurement of Doppler indices.[11,12] With DCI, the umbilical cord can be followed from the fetus to the placental insertion and sampling sites and optimal Doppler angles may be selected with ease (Fig. 7-11). DCI is particularly valuable in tracing the course of the cord when there is oligohydramnios and cord loops are difficult to identify. Arduini et al.[13] have shown that,

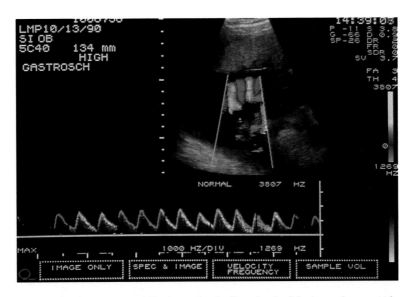

Fig. 7-11 Umbilical artery. Umbilical arteries (red) and vein (blue) are shown with spectral Doppler sample volume positioned within the umbilical artery. The spectral waveform indicates elevation of the systolic/diastolic ratio in this fetus with intrauterine growth retardation.

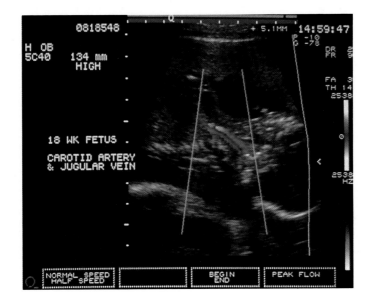

Fig. 7-12 Fetal carotid artery. DCI permits identification of the fetal carotid artery (red) and jugular vein (blue) and aids in selection of site for Doppler sampling.

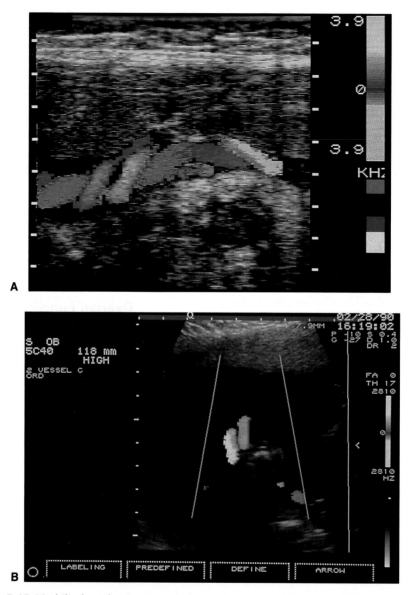

Fig. 7-15 Umbilical cord. **(A)** A normal cord is shown with two umbilical arteries (red) and a single umbilical vein (blue). **(B)** Two-vessel cord with a single umbilical artery. Note the loss of spiral arrangement seen with a normal cord.

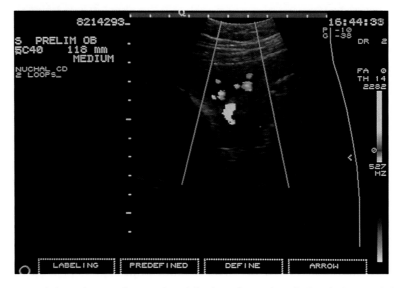

Fig. 7-16 Nuchal cord. Two loops of umbilical cord are identified coiled around the neck of a third-trimester fetus. Two arteries and one vein are shown in each of the loops. The presence of three or more loops is associated with fetal compromise.

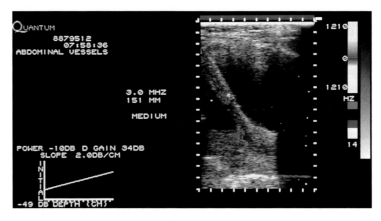

Fig. 7-17 Marginal vein. A low-lying posterior placenta is shown in a third-trimester patient with vaginal bleeding. Prominent vessels are seen near the internal cervical os and were presumed to be the cause of the bleeding.

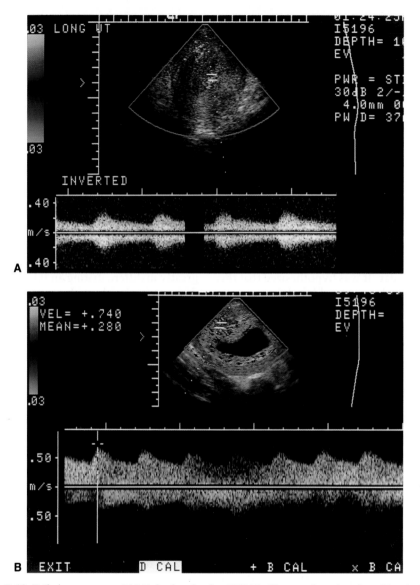

Fig. 7-19 Failed pregnancy. **(A)** Pulsed and color EVUS of incomplete abortion. No obvious products of conception are seen, yet abnormal color flow is noted. Pulsed Doppler shows peak velocities exceeding 25 cm/s and low-impedance flow consistent with placental flow. **(B)** EVUS of blighted ovum showing typical low-impedance and high-velocity placental flow.

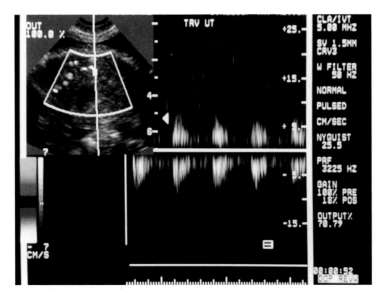

Fig. 7-20 Pseudosac. There is no evidence of the typical pattern of normal placental flow.

to 21 cm/s with an angle of 0 degrees) resulted in misclassification of only 5 of 31 IUP and none of the 9 pseudosacs.

Fibroids

We have demonstrated that because some fibroids may show considerable vascularity, which may be of high velocity and low impedance, they must be differentiated from placental flow (Fig. 7-21). This can best be effected by consideration of the morphologic information. A fibroid is usually associated with myometrial contour deformity, whereas retained products of conception occur in the endometrial cavity. Confusion, however, could theoretically occur with the submucosal fibroid. Consideration of the serum hCG levels in conjunction with the imaging appearance should prevent any confusion in the diagnosis of any vascular masses.

Molar Pregnancy (Gestational Trophoblastic Neoplasia)

Taylor et al.[29] noted the very high velocities and low impedance found in three cases of persistent trophoblastic disease. As with retained products of conception, color Doppler is particularly valuable in demonstrating and localizing this abnormal flow (Fig. 7-22). Although we have been unable to differentiate between retained products of conception and malignant trophoblastic disease in our subsequent observations, the method still has clinical use for the diagnosis and localization of molar disease, especially when this is invasive and appears within the myometrium.

Endometrial Carcinoma

Folkman et al.[30] recognized the importance of angiogenesis in the induction and behavior of malignant tumors. Tumor vessels are ab-

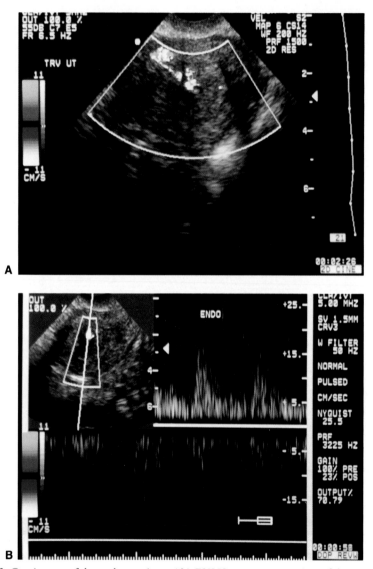

Fig. 7-23 Carcinoma of the endometrium. **(A)** EVUS transverse section of the uterus shows abnormal color flow. **(B)** Pulsed Doppler of this area demonstrates low-impedance flow. In a postmenopausal patient, these appearances are indicative of neovascularization in the endometrium. This patient proved to have carcinoma of the endometrium.

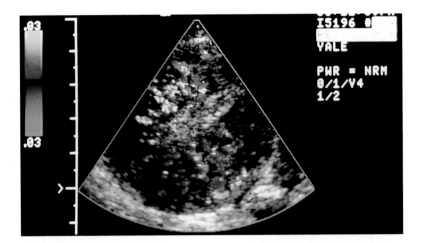

Fig. 7-24 Endometritis. EVUS shows abnormal color flow within the endometrium. Clinically, this patient had pelvic inflammatory disease and proved to have chronic endometritis.

Since ovarian cancer is not a common disease, universal screening for it is unlikely to be cost-effective. Examination of all women over age 50 years would probably disclose one ovarian cancer per thousand. In view of this likelihood, we and others are currently focusing our efforts on screening only patients with a family history of ovarian cancer. Some families have a high familial incidence of cancers of the ovary, breast, and colon and would seem to be worthwhile targets for cost-efficacy studies involving a combination of ultrasound and serum tumor markers. In view of the expected very low positive rate, it is difficult to justify the cost of MRI for screening purposes.

It should be stressed that screening techniques for carcinoma of the ovary, despite their widespread publicity, are essentially experimental protocols. Evaluation of such patients should include a detailed physical examination by an experienced oncologic gynecologist and testing for tumor markers twice per year. In addition, we perform EVUS examinations with color Doppler at 6-month intervals. First, the ovary is carefully examined for abnormality of size or shape. Doppler is then used to search for flow, and flow patterns are characterized by using the time–velocity spectrum derived from the pulsed Doppler. Abnormal ovarian flow is characterized by low-impedance signals in the absence of a corpus luteum.[34] The site of this abnormal flow may be localized expeditiously by the use of color Doppler (Figs. 7-25 and 7-26).

Unfortunately, these criteria lead to many false-positive results. In the premenopausal patient, luteal flow would be identical to that of neovascularization associated with ovarian cancer. It is therefore essential to bring these patients in for examination in the very early part of their cycle, preferably as soon as the menstrual period has ended. Even then, the

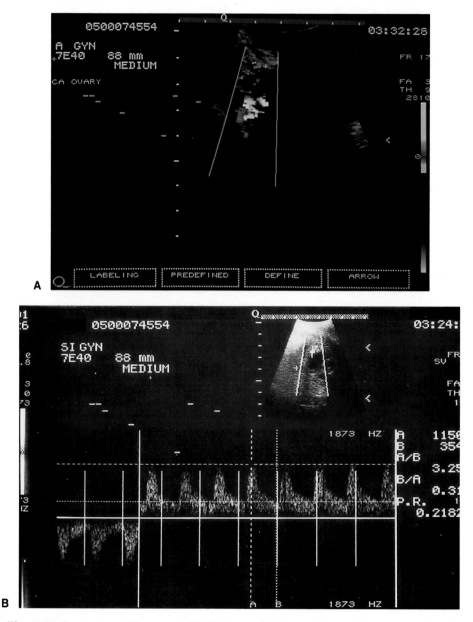

Fig. 7-25 Carcinoma of the ovary. **(A)** DCI reveals abnormal vascularity associated with a complex mass arising from the ovary. **(B)** Doppler spectrum demonstrates low-impedance flow. This finding, although not specific, suggests ovarian cancer.

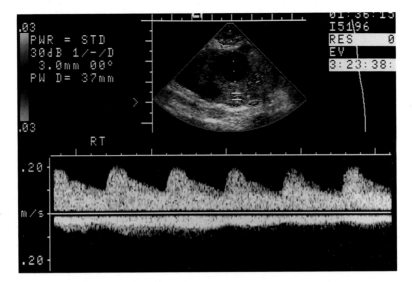

Fig. 7-26 Perimenopausal ovary. Pulsed and color Doppler reveal follicles with abnormal vascularity seen inappropriately early in the cycle. Pulsed Doppler demonstrates low-impedance flow. If this finding persists, it suggests ovarian cancer.

persistence of functional cysts is not uncommon, and if luteal-like flow is demonstrated at that time, the patient should be examined 1 or 3 months later, early in the cycle to see whether this abnormal flow persists. In view of the essentially experimental nature of the Doppler flow investigation, it is unlikely that surgeons would explore a patient with abnormal flow unless the CA125 and other tumor markers were elevated to increase clinical suspicion.

In postmenopausal patients, the situation is less confused by luteal flow. However, for some time after menopause it is possible for functional cysts or even occasional ovulation to occur, and therefore repeated scans and consideration of the tumor marker levels may be necessary before suspicion is raised sufficiently for surgery to be considered.

SUMMARY

The addition of pulsed and color Doppler has greatly added to the diagnostic potential for obstetric and gynecologic ultrasound. In addition to improved morphologic detail inherent in the use of EVUS, new information is available on perfusion and the physiologic changes associated with the menstrual cycle and early pregnancy. The absence of luteal flow strongly predicts unsuccessful pregnancy outcome in patients undergoing therapy for infertility. This introduces the possibility of more economic use of expensive treatments. Later in pregnancy, DCI aids in the efficient and accurate performance of Doppler spectral sampling and contributes to the evaluation of structural and functional abnormalities of the fetus, umbilical cord, and placenta. Applications in the evaluation of patients with suspected ectopic pregnancy, incomplete abortion, and pseudosac are welcome additions for clinical problems that currently result in many malpractice suits. Finally, the recognition of neovascular flow, especially in the ovary, raises hope for improved and earlier diagnosis of ovarian cancer.

REFERENCES

1. American Institute of Ultrasound in Medicine, Bioeffects Committee: Bioeffects considerations for the safety of diagnostic ultrasound. J Ultrasound Med 7(suppl):54, 1988
2. Taylor KJW: A prudent approach to Doppler US. Radiology 165:283, 1987
3. Taylor KJW, Ramos IM, Feyock AL, et al: Ectopic pregnancy: duplex Doppler evaluation. Radiology 173:93, 1989
4. Campbell S, Griffin DR, Pearce JM, et al: New Doppler technique for assessing uteroplacental blood flow. Lancet 1:675, 1983
5. Schulman H, Fleischer A, Farmakides G, et al: Development of uterine artery compliance in pregnancy as detected by Doppler ultrasound. Am J Obstet Gynecol 155:1031, 1986
6. Brosens I, Robertson WB, Dixon HG: The physiological response of the vessels of the placental bed to normal pregnancy. J Pathol Bacteriol 93:569, 1967
7. Dillon E, Feyock AL, Taylor KJW: Pseudogestational sacs: Doppler US differentiation from normal or abnormal intrauterine pregnancies. Radiology 176:359, 1990
8. Carroll BA: Duplex Doppler systems in obstetric ultrasound. Radiol Clin North Am 28:189, 1990
9. Tyrrell S, Obaid AH, Lilford RJ: Umbilical artery Doppler velocimetry as a predictor of fetal hypoxia and acidosis at birth. Obstet Gynecol 74:332, 1989
10. Gaziano E, Knox GE, Wager GP, et al: The predictability of the small-for-gestational-age infant by real-time ultrasound-derived measurements combined with pulsed Doppler umbilical artery velocimetry. Am J Obstet Gynecol 158:1431, 1988
11. Maulik D, Yarlagadda AP, Youngblood JP,
Willoughby L: Components of variability of umbilical arterial Doppler velocimetry—a prospective analysis. Am J Obstet Gynecol 160:1406, 1989
12. Kay HH, Carroll BA, Bowie JD, et al: Nonuniformity of fetal umbilical systolic/diastolic ratios as determined with duplex Doppler sonography. J Ultrasound Med 8:417, 1989
13. Arduini D, Rizzo G, Boccolini MR, et al: Functional assessment of uteroplacental and fetal circulations by means of color Doppler ultrasonography. J Ultrasound Med 9:249, 1990
14. Jauniaux E, Campbell S, Vyas S: The use of color Doppler imaging for prenatal diagnosis of umbilical cord anomalies: report of three cases. Am J Obstet Gyncol 161:1195, 1989
15. Birnholz JC: Ecologic physiology of the fetus. Ultrasonography of supply-line deprivation syndromes. Radiol Clin North Am 28:179, 1990
16. DeVore GR, Horenstein J, Siassi B, Platt LD: Fetal echocardiography. VII. Doppler color flow mapping: a new technique for the diagnosis of congenital heart disease. Am J Obstet Gynecol 156:1054, 1987
17. Chiba Y, Kanzaki T, Kobayashi H, et al: Evaluation of fetal structural heart disease using color flow mapping. Ultrasound Med Biol 16:221, 1990
18. DiSessa TG, Emerson DS, Felker RE, et al: Anomalous systemic and pulmonary venous pathways diagnosed in utero by ultrasound. J Ultrasound Med 9:311, 1990
19. Harding JA, Lewis DF, Major CA, et al: Color flow Doppler—a useful instrument in the diagnosis of vasa previa. Am J Obstet Gynecol 163:1566, 1990
20. Nelson LH, Melone PJ, King M: Diagnosis of vasa previa with transvaginal and color flow Doppler ultrasound. Obstet Gynecol 76:506, 1990
21. Taylor KJW, Burns PN, Wells PNT, et al: Ultrasound Doppler flow studies of the ovarian and uterine arteries. Br J Obstet Gynaecol 92:240, 1985
22. Deutinger J, Reinthaller A, Bernaschek: Transvaginal pulsed Doppler measurement of blood flow velocity in the ovarian arteries during cycle stimulation and after follicle puncture. Fertil Steril 51:466, 1989

23. Hata K, Hata T, Senoh D, et al: Change in ovarian arterial compliance during the human menstrual cycle assessed by Doppler ultrasound. Br J Obstet Gynaecol 97:163, 1990

24. Baber RJ, McSweeney MB, Gill RW, et al: Transvaginal pulsed Doppler ultrasound assessment of blood flow to the corpus luteum in IVF patients following embryo transfer. Br J Obstet Gynaecol 95:1226, 1988

25. Russell JB, Lambert J, Taylor KJW, DeCherney AH: Androgen-producing hilus cell tumor of the ovary: detection in a postmenopausal woman by duplex Doppler scanning. JAMA 257:962, 1987

26. Pellerito J, Case C, Hammers L, et al: Transvaginal color Doppler flow imaging in the evaluation of ectopic pregnancy. Radiology 177:117, 1990

27. Myers MT: Duplex Doppler and transvaginal sonography for the evaluation of ectopic pregnancy. M.D. Thesis. Yale University, New Haven, CT, 1989

28. Bradley WG, Fiske CE, Filly RA: The double sac sign of early intrauterine pregnancy: use in exclusion of ectopic pregnancy. Radiology 143:223, 1982

29. Taylor KJW, Schwartz PE, Kohorn EI: Gestational trophoblastic neoplasia: diagnosis with Doppler US. Radiology 165:445, 1987

30. Folkman J, Watson K, Ingber D, Hanahan D: Induction of angiogenesis during the transition from hyperplasia to neoplasia. Nature 339:58, 1989

31. Taylor KJW, Ramos I, Carter D, et al: Correlation of Doppler US tumor signals with neovascular morphologic features. Radiology 166:57, 1988

32. Bourne TH, Campbell S, Whitehead MI, et al: Detection of endometrial cancer in post menopausal women by transvaginal ultrasonography and colour flow imaging. Br Med J 301:369, 1990

33. Kurjak A, Zalud I, Alfirevic Z, Jurkovic D: The assessment of abnormal blood flow by transvaginal color and pulse Doppler. Ultrasound Med Biol 16:437, 1990

34. Bourne TH, Campbell C, Steer V, et al: Transvaginal colour flow imaging—a new screening technique for ovarian cancer. Br Med J 299:1367, 1989

8

Scrotum, Breast, Thyroid, and Extremities

David M. Paushter
Gregory P. Borkowski

Ultrasound of small parts refers to the evaluation of superficial body parts by using high-frequency transducers. Included in this group of body parts are the thyroid and parathyroid glands, other neck masses, the scrotum, the penis, the breast, and other palpable, superficial vascular and nonvascular masses. The imaging and color Doppler demands of small-parts sonography frequently differ from those of abdominal or pelvic examinations by virtue of the superficial location of the abnormality being studied. This chapter reviews the utility of Doppler color imaging (DCI) when applied to small-parts sonography with special emphasis on technologic and scanning requirements.

INSTRUMENTATION AND TECHNICAL CONSIDERATIONS

There is great variability in the currently available color Doppler equipment in terms of both acquisition and display of Doppler-shifted frequency information. A primary requirement of small-parts DCI is high sensitivity to slow-flow states. This is frequently needed because of the small size of the vessels being evaluated and the associated minimal blood flow velocities. Although some manufacturers claim sensitivity to velocities as low as 0.3 cm/s, in practice it is difficult for the user to evaluate such a statement objectively, since flow sensitivity is dependent on multiple factors including transducer Doppler frequency, frame rate, filters, persistence functions, vessel size, and vessel depth. Regardless of the equipment, it is important to set the color gain velocity scale and dwell time appropriately for the expected flow pattern and velocities being evaluated. A cineloop function is extremely useful in small-parts scanning, since minute vessels and associated flow patterns may be very difficult to evaluate by image freezing.

Although higher transducer frequency improves sensitivity to slow flow, it may result in color Doppler aliasing when the Doppler-shifted frequency exceeds the Nyquist frequency of the transducer. Aliasing can be overcome by changing the color scale, increasing the Doppler angle, or utilizing a lower-frequency transducer. Other commonly encountered artifacts include "bleeding" of vessel color into the surrounding soft tissues as a result of inadequate optimization of gray-scale and color priorities.[1,2] False color information may occur in anechoic fluid collections, particularly if echo intensity is utilized to suppress color.[1,3] This type of color information may be separated from true flow, since it appears to be random and represents noise when spectral Doppler tracings are obtained.

In addition to these artifacts, a visible bruit may be identified adjacent to larger vessels as a result of transmitted pulsations.[1,2,4] Although this may interfere with image interpretation, at times it may also suggest the existence of a vascular abnormality, such as a stenosis, which requires evaluation of adjacent arteries and veins. A mirror-image artifact may occur deep to large arteries.[1,4,5] This can be avoided by changing the scanning angle or possibly reducing the Doppler gain. Finally, wall filters that are meant to diminish low-amplitude signals from vessel wall motion may obscure diastolic flow, particularly within small vessels. When this information is required, adjustable wall filters must be set as low as possible.

SCROTUM

Testicular scintigraphy has been the mainstay for the evaluation of the acute scrotum, with an accuracy of approximately 90 to 95 percent in the diagnosis of testicular torsion.[6–8] Recently, DCI has been applied to the evaluation of the acute scrotum as well.[9–13]

The ability to detect scrotal blood flow, par-

ticularly in the intratesticular arteries, is dependent on equipment sensitivity to slow-flow states. In particular, units utilizing a Doppler frequency of 7.5 MHz will have an improved signal-to-noise ratio compared with 5-MHz transducers, because of an increase in Doppler-shifted frequencies from the red blood cells. With resultant equipment variation in terms of flow sensitivity, it is prudent to evaluate a series of normal testicles before formulating guidelines for absence of flow. Similarly, during acute scrotal evaluation, comparison with the contralateral, uninvolved testicle will aid in providing an internal control.

Depending on equipment flow sensitivity, supratesticular and capsular arteries are most frequently visualized (Fig. 8-1).[9] Intratesticular arteries are also frequently seen, demonstrating a low-resistance waveform and peak systolic velocity averaging slightly less than 10 cm/s. Intratesticular arteries include the centripital arteries and recurrent rami. When coursing through the mediastinum testis, the testicular artery frequently does not penetrate to the opposite free testicular surface, and the accompanying testicular vein may be imaged.

There is some variation in the literature on the criteria necessary for diagnosis of testicular torsion. Utilizing absence of intratesticular arteries, the technique has been reported to have a sensitivity of 86 percent and a specificity of 100 percent,[11] whereas utilizing the criterion of no flow in the affected testicle compared with flow in the contralateral testicle or skin on the affected side, a sensitivity and specificity of 100 percent have been obtained for the diagnosis of torsion.[12] More recently, it has been suggested that absent or "dramatically reduced" flow compared with the contralateral normal testicle may be the most appropriate criterion.[13]

In acute testicular torsion there is usually no

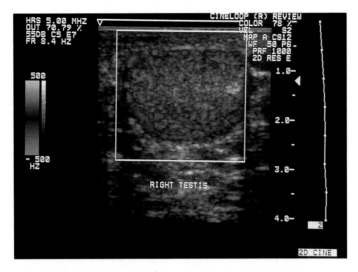

Fig. 8-1 Normal testicle. Longitudinal ultrasound image demonstrates peripheral flow around a normal testicle on this 5-MHz examination. A few central arteries are also visualized.

accompanying peritesticular increased flow, whereas this is frequently seen with chronic torsion. Similarly, in patients who have undergone spontaneous or manipulative detorsion, flow to the affected testicle may be normal or increased.[11] Appendiceal torsion results in normal testicular flow but frequently an increase in peritesticular vasculature.[11,13] As expected, increased flow is commonly identified when there is inflammatory change in the epididymis or testicle.[11,13]

There is no published information on the utility of DCI in the evaluation of the non-acute scrotum. We have examined an array of testicular masses by this technique and in the majority of instances have been unable to demonstrate other than minimal flow within testicular neoplasms or abscesses (Fig. 8-2). We have, however, demonstrated flow within an extratesticular, intrascrotal metastasis, allowing differentiation from a complex cystic mass such as a spermatocele (Fig. 8-3).

A varicocele represents tortuous, dilated veins of the pampiniform plexus, usually in the left hemiscrotum. Varicoceles may be painful, occasionally are associated with cancer, and are a common cause of infertility. Ultrasound imaging has been used for diagnosis, as have non-Doppler ultrasound, radioisotope scanning, and venography. Ultrasound imaging demonstrates multiple tortuous, tubular structures adjacent to the superior pole of the testicle. The varicocele increases in size with the Valsalva maneuver or upright posture and, at times, venous flow can be visually identified.[14]

Duplex sonography can quickly establish the diagnosis of varicocele by demonstrating venous flow within these dilated channels. Similarly, we use DCI to demonstrate the vascular nature of these abnormalities (Fig. 8-4). This allows differentiation from other complex cystic structures in this region, such as spermatocele, in a rapid, conclusive manner. Slowing or cessation of flow within the varicocele and associated dilatation can also

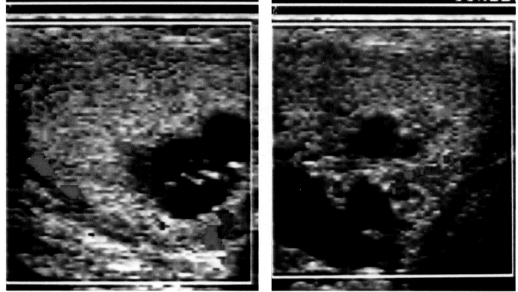

A   B

Fig. 8-2 Testicular abscess. **(A)** Longitudinal and **(B)** transverse ultrasound images demonstrate a hypoechoic testicular mass with internal septations. Peripheral testicular flow is present with vessels approaching the abscess as well.

be identified with the Valsalva maneuver and upright position.

BREAST

In women, breast cancer is the most frequent neoplasm encountered and the second leading cause of cancer death.[15] Currently, mammography is the most sensitive imaging modality available for detection and characterization of breast masses. Although mammography is highly sensitive for detection of masses, it has a limited ability to differentiate various types of breast lesions. Historically, the role of ultrasound in this regard has been to distinguish cystic from solid masses within the breast.

Taylor et al.[16] have identified abnormal Doppler signals obtained by duplex sonography in a variety of malignant tumors. The most common tumor signal obtained was a high-velocity shift suggestive of arteriovenous shunting; this was present in 86 percent of 44 patients examined. In 20 percent of these patients, an almost continuous, high-velocity Doppler-shifted frequency was obtained.

Duplex sonography has also been applied to the evaluation of breast masses. Schoenberger et al.[17] evaluated 38 solid breast masses by duplex sonography without DCI. They were able to obtain a waveform or audible signal in all 12 patients with infiltrative ductal carcinoma but in none of the 26 with benign conditions. The signal was obtained from the peripheral portion of the mass or interface with normal breast tissue and was unrelated to the size of the mass. No Doppler signals could be obtained from the contralateral, normal breast. The waveform obtained from the carcinomas was that of a low-resistance

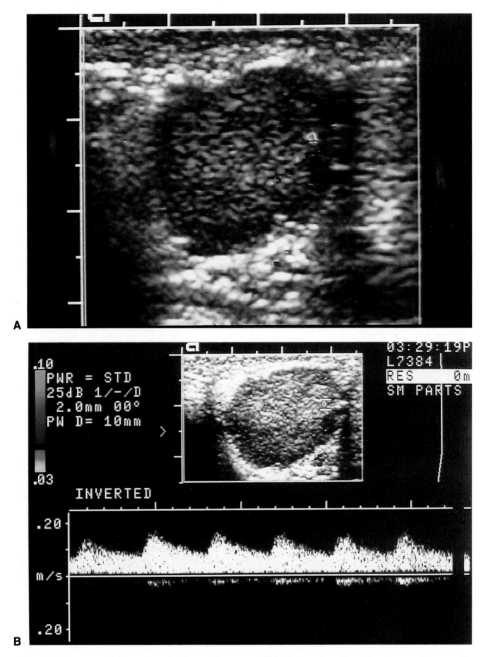

Fig. 8-3 Metastatic, extratesticular melanoma. **(A)** This color Doppler image shows a hypoechoic mass with internal vasculature. **(B)** Spectral Doppler tracing demonstrates a low-resistance arterial waveform.

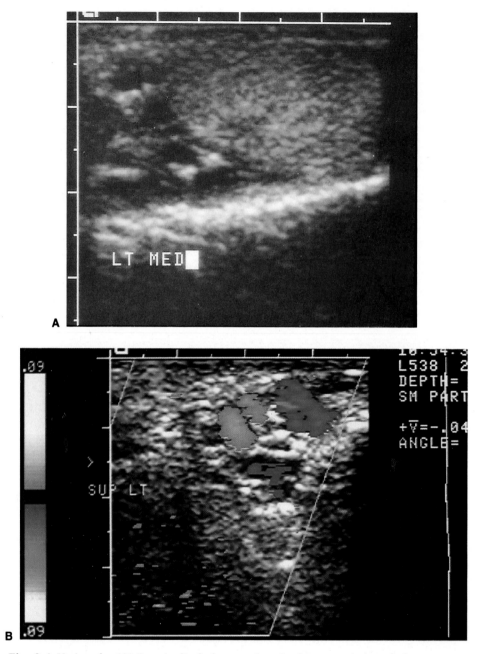

Fig. 8-4 Varicocele. **(A)** Longitudinal ultrasound study shows anechoic, tubular structures adjacent to the cranial testicle. **(B)** Color Doppler image demonstrates internal flow characteristics of varicocele, which is corroborated by the **(C)** spectral tracing. (*Figure continues.*)

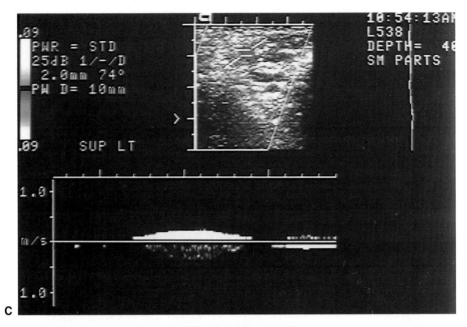

Fig. 8-4 (*Continued*).

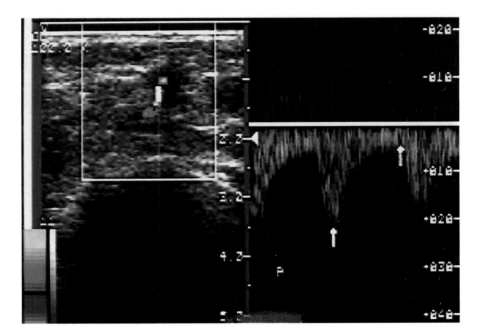

Fig. 8-5 Medullary carcinoma of the breast. Color Doppler examination demonstrates central flow within a hypoechoic breast mass with associated arterial tracing by spectral analysis.

breast masses remains a research tool. Current information does not suggest that carcinoma can be differentiated from benign masses sufficiently accurately to direct biopsy.

MALE IMPOTENCE

During the last decade, it has been determined that most cases of impotence have an organic etiology. This has spurred the search for newer, noninvasive diagnostic techniques including duplex sonography with DCI to evaluate arterial and venous insufficiency.

Since the original description of penile duplex techniques by Lue et al.,[20] several authors have utilized conventional duplex and DCI in an attempt to identify arteriogenic impotence.[21-25] These studies have frequently suffered from a lack of correlative angiographic data. This technique involves duplex sampling of the paired cavernosal arteries within the corpora cavernosa after intracavernosal injection of vasoactive drugs such as papaverine, phentolamine, or prostaglandin E_1. DCI has been used for improved visualization of these small arteries and appropriate angle correction for velocity measurements. Owing to the small size of the cavernosal arteries and low velocities encountered, the sensitivity of the ultrasound unit to slow flow is critical.

Approximately 5 minutes after intracavernosal drug injection, angle-corrected peak

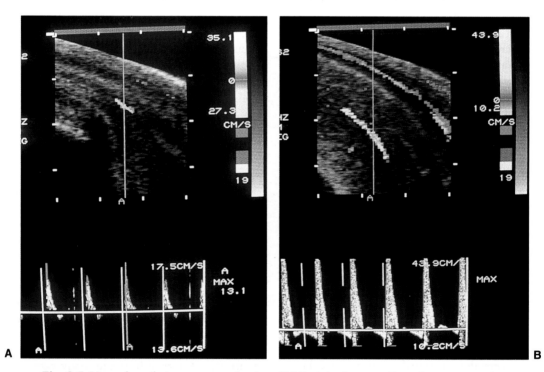

Fig. 8-7 Normal penile impotence evaluation. **(A)** Preinjection waveform demonstrates the small size of the cavernosal artery with high-resistance, low-amplitude waveform. **(B)** Seven minutes after injection, the cavernosal artery has increased markedly in size. Peak systolic velocity is approximately 50 cm/s with negative end-diastolic flow.

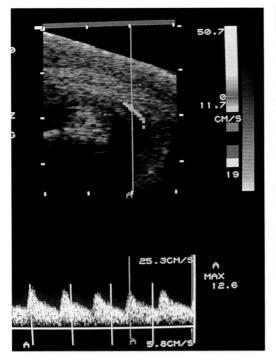

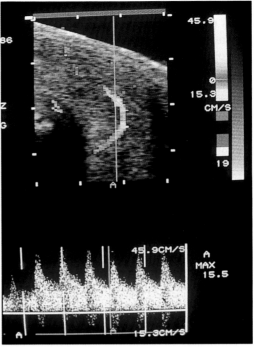

Fig. 8-8 Arteriogenic impotence. This tracing, obtained 5 minutes after injection, shows peak systolic velocity of only 12.6 cm/s, consistent with arterial insufficiency.

Fig. 8-9 Venogenic impotence. Spectral Doppler tracing 6 minutes after injection demonstrates an end-diastolic velocity of 15.5 cm/s, consistent with venous leak.

systolic velocity measurements are obtained from the cavernosal arteries (Fig. 8-7). Repeated readings at 1-minute intervals for an additional 5 minutes may be needed to obtain the highest-velocity readings. Although criteria for diagnosis of arteriogenic impotence have varied,[21,22,23,24] certainly patients with peak systolic velocities less than 25 cm/s are likely to have arterial insufficiency. We consider velocity readings of 25 to 30 cm/s a "gray zone," with readings above 30 cm/s within the normal range (Fig. 8-8). In addition, it has been suggested that asymmetric peak systolic velocities in the right and left cavernosal arteries may be indicative of mild to moderate arterial disease.[23]

The cavernosal artery waveform can also provide important information on venogenic impotence.[22,24] Engagement of the penile veno-occlusive mechanism results in increased resistance to arterial in-flow with concomitant changes in the diastolic portion of the cavernosal artery waveform. It has been suggested that an end-diastolic velocity greater than 5 cm/s is indicative of a venous leak,[24] and our results agree with this conclusion[26] (Fig. 8-9). We have, however, found that it may be necessary to obtain repeated Doppler tracings for up to 15 minutes after drug injection to obtain this information. We have also determined that an end-diastolic velocity consistently 2 cm/s or lower is highly suggestive of a normal veno-occlusive mechanism.

The technique of evaluation of vasculogenic impotence by DCI requires meticulous Doppler sampling, accurate Doppler angle determination, and attention to anatomic

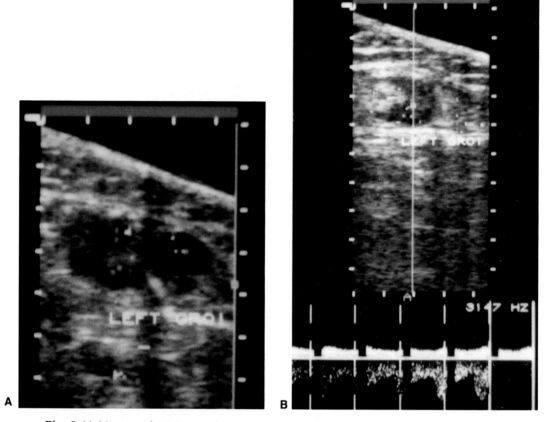

Fig. 8-11 Non-neoplastic inguinal lymph node. **(A)** Small vessels radiating from the nodal hilum are identified on this color Doppler image. **(B)** Spectral Doppler tracing demonstrates arterial and venous flow within the lymph node.

and major vascular encasement by tumor. Compression of the internal jugular vein by lymph node metastasis can be demonstrated, as can thrombosis.

DCI allows visualization of the internal architecture of the normal lymph node, including a hilum, with a central artery and vein having internal branches (Fig. 8-11).[32,33] Although little information is available in this regard, it appears that the internal architecture is more likely to be preserved with benign lymphadenopathy than with malignant involvement.[33] Further studies are necessary to determine whether lymphoma can be accurately distinguished from benign lymphadenopathy by identification of straightening of nodal vessels. We have used DCI to determine the effects of cervical nodal masses on the carotid artery and jugular vein (Fig. 8-12), and it is likely that direct vascular invasion may be more easily visualized by this technique than by ultrasound imaging alone.

Evaluation of other spontaneous or post-traumatic masses by DCI may provide im-

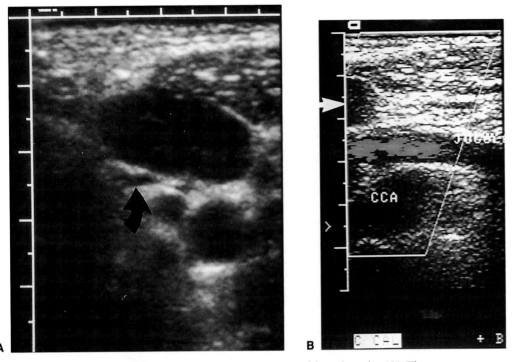

A   **B**

Fig. 8-12 Squamous cell carcinoma metastatic to cervical lymph node. **(A)** The transverse ultrasound image shows a large nodal mass anterior to the compressed jugular vein (curved arrow) and carotid branches. **(B)** Longitudinal color Doppler image demonstrates a minimal, blue flow stream adjacent to the nodal mass (arrow).

portant information without the need to resort to angiography for diagnosis. Conventional duplex sonography and DCI have been demonstrated to accurately portray vascular abnormalities such as pseudoaneurysms and arteriovenous fistulae.[34–42] Although the majority of these abnormalities are the result of known vascular injury due to arterial catheterization or previous vascular surgery, patients will occasionally present with them with minimal or no history of trauma (Fig. 8-13). DCI allows quick and accurate assessment of such masses and distinguishes them from solid masses, hematomas, abscesses, and lymphoceles.

The technique of evaluation of a peripheral mass is initiated by using ultrasound imaging for determination of echotexture. DCI techniques are then employed for display of intrinsic vascularity. With false aneurysms (Fig. 8-14), the tract leading from the adjacent artery is often visualized and Doppler sampling will demonstrate the typical "to-and-fro" motion of the blood entering and exiting the pseudoaneurysm.[34,35,37,38,41,42]

Similarly, in arteriovenous fistulas, the communication between the adjacent arteries and vein is often visualized.[36,39,40,41] Persistent intra-arterial flow in diastole and associated

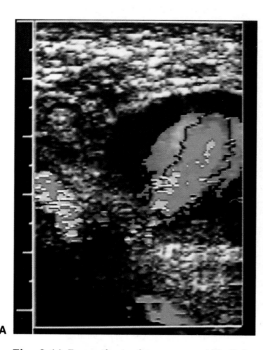

A

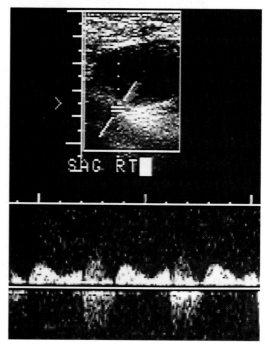

B

Fig. 8-14 Femoral pseudoaneurysm. **(A)** Color Doppler longitudinal image demonstrates turbulent flow with associated peripheral thrombus within a large groin collection. **(B)** The tract connecting this pseudoaneurysm with the femoral artery is well identified on the second image. **(C)** There is oscillation of flow above and below the baseline on the spectral Doppler tracing.

C

venous turbulence are present. Pulsatile flow may be recorded with Doppler spectral sampling in the adjacent vein.

Other vascular anomalies such as superficial varices, venous aneurysms, and cutaneous hemangiomata can be evaluated by DCI (Figs. 8-15 and 8-16). This may corroborate the suspected etiology of the mass and provide additional information. We have also

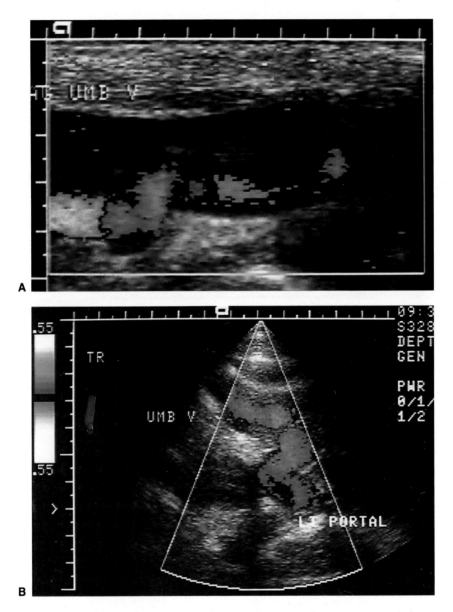

Fig. 8-15 Patent umbilical vein. **(A)** Color Doppler image demonstrates a tubular, ectatic vein in the subcutaneous tissues. **(B)** This could be traced to the left portal vein in this patient with cirrhosis and portal hypertension.

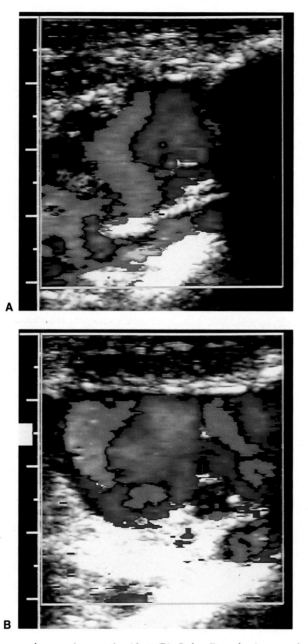

Fig. 8-16 Cutaneous hemangiomatosis. **(A & B)** Color Doppler images show dilated, vascular channels in the subcutaneous tissues, consistent with hemangiomatosis. Venous tracings were obtained.

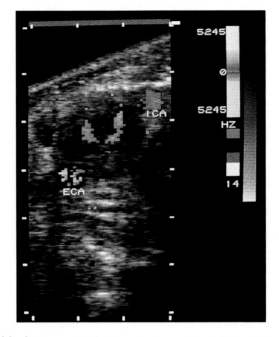

Fig. 8-17 Carotid body tumor. Radiating arteries are identified within this paraganglioma between the internal (ICA) and external (ECA) carotid arteries on this transverse color Doppler image.

found DCI useful in the evaluation of masses that are not primarily vascular (Fig. 8-17). Occasionally, the intrinsic vasculature of solid masses may make them more conspicuous and even suggest a diagnosis.[43] In addition, assessment of relative tumor vascularity may aid in biopsy planning. Fine-needle aspiration may be preferred to large-bore, cutting-needle biopsy if DCI demonstrates abundant vascularity.

ORBIT

Few articles have addressed the potential utility of DCI in the evaluation of orbital vascular abnormalities. Erickson et al.,[44] utilizing a 7.5-MHz imaging and Doppler transducer, found that a "slow-flow" package

could not be used because of ocular motion. They were able to visualize the ophthalmic artery and its central retinal and posterior ciliary branches in 26 normal orbits. There was 100 percent visualization of the central retinal vein and venae vorticosae as well. The terminal lacrimal artery and superior ophthalmic vein were visualized in 19 and 22 of 26 normal orbits, respectively. The supratrochlear and supraorbital arteries were difficult to image, and the inferior ophthalmic vein was not seen.

Erickson et al.[44] were able to identify carotid-cavernous fistula by observing enlargement of the superior ophthalmic vein (Fig. 8-18) with "arterialized" reversed flow. There was also reversed flow in the supraorbital vein. Similarly, single cases of orbital varix and arteriovenous malformation were also visu-

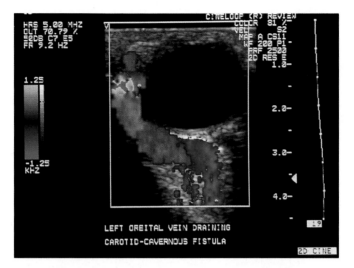

Fig. 8-18 Carotid-cavernous fistula. Color Doppler study shows enlarged, tortuous ophthalmic vein.

alized. A diagnosis of superior ophthalmic vein thrombosis was made by lack of visualization of a patent vein and apparent venous collaterals. Nonvascular masses involving the orbit were also imaged and therefore could be separated from masses with other vascular etiologies.

SUMMARY

DCI, when coupled with small-parts grayscale imaging, has demonstrated great utility in the evaluation of superficial body abnormalities. This technique has rapidly become a primary method of evaluation of suspected testicular torsion, and its results are competitive with those of standard nuclear medicine examinations. DCI evaluation of male impotence, coupled with intracavernous injection of vasoactive substances, is now a leading, noninvasive technique for diagnosis of both arteriogenic and venogenic causes. DCI may provide invaluable information in the evaluation of palpable masses, particularly in the diagnosis of vascular abnormalities such as false aneurysm and arteriovenous fistula.

Further studies are needed to corroborate the utility of DCI in the evaluation of focal thyroid and parathyroid abnormalities, breast carcinoma, nodal cancer, and the orbit. Because this technique is applicable to superficial, high-frequency examinations, DCI is rapidly becoming an accepted and frequently necessary part of any small-parts ultrasound study.

REFERENCES

1. Mitchell DG: Color Doppler imaging: principles, limitations, and artifacts. Radiology 177:1, 1990
2. Foley WD, Erickson SJ: Color Doppler flow imaging. AJR 156:3, 1991
3. Mitchell DG, Burns P, Needleman L: Color Doppler artifact in anechoic regions. J Ultrasound Med 9:255, 1990

4. Middleton WD, Melson GL: The carotid ghost: a color Doppler ultrasound duplication artifact. J Ultrasound Med 9:487, 1990
5. Middleton WD, Erickson S, Melson GL: Perivascular color artifact: pathologic significance and appearance on color Doppler US images. Radiology 171:647, 1989
6. Chen DCP, Holder LE, Kaplan GN: Correlation of radionuclide imaging and diagnostic ultrasound in scrotal diseases. J Nuclear Med 27:1774, 1986
7. Haynes BE, Bessen HA, Haynes VE: The diagnosis of testicular torsion. JAMA 18:2522, 1983
8. Chen DCP, Holder LE, Melloul M: Radionuclide scrotal imaging: further experience with 210 patients—results and discussion. J Nuclear Med 25(pt 2):841, 1983
9. Middleton WD, Thorne DA, Melson GL: Color Doppler ultrasound of the normal testis. AJR 152:293, 1989
10. Middleton WD, Melson GL: Testicular ischemia: color Doppler sonographic findings in five patients. AJR 152:1237, 1989
11. Burks DD, Markey BJ, Burkhard TK, et al: Suspected testicular torsion and ischemia: evaluation with color Doppler sonography. Radiology 175:815, 1990
12. Lerner RM, Mevorach RA, Hulbert WC, Rabinowitz R: Color Doppler US in the evaluation of acute scrotal disease. Radiology 176:355, 1990
13. Middleton WD, Siegel BA, Melson GL, et al: Acute scrotal disorders: prospective comparison of color Doppler US and testicular scintigraphy. Radiology 177:177, 1990
14. Wolverson MK, Hourttuin E, Heiberg E, et al: High-resolution real-time sonography of scrotal varicocele. AJR 141:775, 1983
15. Boring CC, Squires TS, Tony T: Cancer statistics, 1991. CA-a Cancer J Clin 41(1):19, 1991
16. Taylor KJW, Ramos I, Carter D, et al: Correlation of Doppler US tumor signals with neovascular morphologic features. Radiology 166:57, 1988
17. Schoenberger SG, Sutherland CM, Robinson AE: Breast neoplasms: duplex sonographic imaging as an adjunct in diagnosis. Radiology 168:665, 1988
18. Jackson VP: Breast neoplasms: duplex sonographic imaging as an adjunct in diagnoses (Letter). Radiology 170:578, 1989
19. Cosgrove DO, Bamber JC, Davey JB, et al: Color Doppler signals from breast tumors. Radiology 176:175, 1990
20. Lue TF, Hricak H, Marich KW, Tanagho EA: Vasculogenic impotence evaluated by high-resolution ultrasonography and pulsed Doppler spectrum analysis. Radiology 155:777, 1985
21. Krysiewicz S, Mellinger BC: The role of imaging in the diagnostic evaluation of impotence. AJR 153:1133, 1989
22. Quam JP, King BF, James EM, et al: Duplex and color Doppler sonographic evaluation of vasculogenic impotence. AJR 153:1141, 1989
23. Benson CB, Vickers MA: Sexual impotence caused by vascular disease: diagnosis with duplex sonography. AJR 153:1149, 1989
24. Schwartz AN, Wang KY, Mack LA, et al: Evaluation of normal erectile function with color flow Doppler sonography. AJR 153:1155, 1989
25. Paushter DM: Role of duplex sonography in the evaluation of sexual impotence. AJR 153:1161, 1989
26. Paushter DM, Robertson S, Hale J, et al: Venogenic impotence: evaluation with color flow Doppler. Radiology 177(suppl):177, 1990
27. Ralls PW, Mayekawa DS, Lee KP, et al: Color-flow Doppler sonography in Graves disease: "thyroid inferno". AJR 150:781, 1988
28. Krubsack AJ, Wilson SD, Lawson TL, et al: Prospective comparison of radionuclide computed tomographic, sonographic and magnetic resonance localization of parathyroid tumors. Surgery 106:639, 1989
29. Hajek PC, Salomonowitz E, Turk R, et al: Lymph nodes of the neck: evaluation with US. Radiology 158:739, 1986
30. Majer MC, Hess CF, Kolbel G, Schmiedl U: Small arteries in peripheral lymph nodes: a specific US sign of lymphomatous involvement. Radiology 168:241, 1988
31. Gritzmann N, Grasl MC, Helmer M, Steiner E: Invasion of the carotid artery and jugular vein by lymph node metastases: detection with sonography. AJR 154:411, 1990
32. Morton MJ, Charboneau JW, Banks PM: In-

guinal lymphadenopathy simulating a false aneurysm on color-flow Doppler sonography. AJR 151:115, 1988

33. Liu J, Merton DA, Mitchell DG, et al: Color Doppler imaging of the iliofemoral region. RadioGraphics 10:403, 1990

34. Mitchell DG, Needleman L, Bezzi M, et al: Femoral artery pseudoaneurysm: diagnosis with conventional duplex and color Doppler US. Radiology 165:687, 1987

35. Coughlin BF, Paushter DM: Peripheral pseudoaneurysms: evaluation with duplex US. Radiology 168:339, 1988

36. Igidbashian VN, Mitchell DG, Middleton WD, et al: Iatrogenic femoral arteriovenous fistula: diagnosis with color Doppler imaging. Radiology 170:749, 1989

37. Middleton WD, Picus DD, Marx MV, Melson GL: Color Doppler sonography of hemodialysis vascular access: comparison with angiography. AJR 152:633, 1989

38. Polak JF, Donaldson MC, Whittemore AD, et al: Pulsatile masses surrounding vascular prostheses: real-time US color flow imaging. Radiology 170:363, 1989

39. Helvie MA, Rubin J: Evaluation of traumatic groin arteriovenous fistulas with duplex Doppler sonography. J Ultrasound Med 8:21, 1989

40. Sacks D, Robinson ML, Perlmutter GS: Femoral arterial injury following catheterization: duplex evaluation. J Ultrasound Med 8:241, 1989

41. Roubidoux MA, Hertzberg BS, Carroll BA, Hedgepeth CA: Color flow and image-directed Doppler ultrasound evaluation of iatrogenic arteriovenous fistulas in the groin. J Clin Ultrasound 18:463, 1990

42. Helvie MA, Rubin JM, Silver TM, Kresowik TF: The distinction between femoral artery pseudoaneurysms and other causes of groin masses: value of duplex Doppler sonography. AJR 150:1177, 1988

43. Shulak JF, O'Donovan PB, Paushter DM, Lanzieri CF: Color flow Doppler of carotid body paraganglioma. J Ultrasound Med 8:519, 1989

44. Erickson SJ, Hendrix LE, Massaro BM, et al: Color Doppler flow imaging of the normal and abnormal orbit. Radiology 173:511, 1989

9

Intraoperative and Cranial Applications

Christopher R. B. Merritt

Although the major impact of Doppler color imaging (DCI) has been in peripheral vascular and abdominal applications, the versatility and power of this form of ultrasound have encouraged its use in a number of specialized settings. These include a variety of intraoperative uses and the evaluation of intracranial blood flow in infants. The use of DCI for transcranial Doppler is also emerging as a potentially valuable method.

INTRAOPERATIVE DOPPLER COLOR IMAGING

The contribution of ultrasound in the operating room might be questioned since the surgeon has the opportunity for direct evaluation of the structures of interest. Yet despite precise preoperative localization of abnormalities by using ultrasound, computed tomography (CT), and magnetic resonance imaging (MRI), there are many situations in which the surgeon is unable to ascertain the location and nature of deep-seated abnormalities by direct inspection and palpation at the time of surgery. Information about the

vascularity of both normal and abnormal structures may be invaluable to the surgeon in making decisions related to surgical management. This need for additional information at the time of operation has stimulated attempts to improve intraoperative localization. Stereotactic approaches utilizing radiography and CT have been devised for operative localization for certain procedures, particularly involving the central nervous system (CNS); however, these devices are expensive and cumbersome. Intraoperative CT has also been described, but it is impractical for most hospitals. In almost all cases, ultrasound is capable of providing real-time intraoperative guidance for operative localization, rendering these more complex and costly approaches unnecessary. The addition of flow imaging to the tissue-imaging capabilities of intraoperative ultrasound significantly extends its range of applications.

The operative environment is ideal for the use of ultrasound. Direct scanning on the organ of interest permits use of high-frequency, high-resolution scanners, and problems caused by interposed gas and bone are

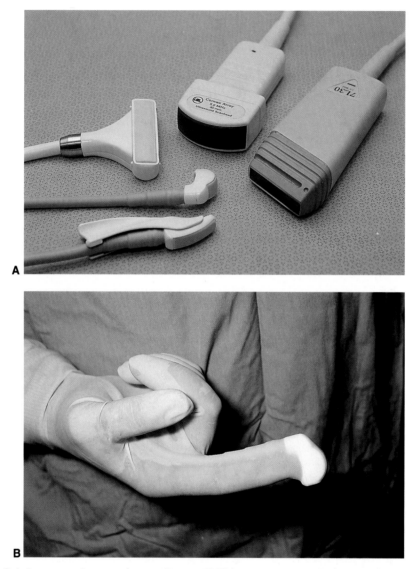

Fig. 9-1 Intraoperative transducers. Current DCI instruments permit the use of a variety of transducers. **(A)** Shown in clockwise fashion from 12 o'clock are a 5.0-MHz curved array (Advanced Technology Laboratories), a 7.5-MHz linear array (Quantum Medical Systems), and special-purpose 3.0- to 7.5-MHz probes (Hitachi Medical Systems) used for intraoperative scanning in our department. **(B)** Some probes may be worn within the ultrasonographer's glove, permitting excellent access to structures of interest, particularly in the abdomen and pelvis.

eliminated.[1,2] As is true elsewhere, the addition of information related to blood flow provided by DCI complements the results of imaging and simple duplex Doppler, thereby enhancing the value of the examination. By facilitating the surgery, operative ultrasound reduces the length of the procedure and results in fewer operative complications. In some cases, imaging alone is adequate to provide the surgeon with information related to the location of an abnormality and its relationship to normal anatomic structures. In other cases, however, the identification of normal and abnormal blood vessels is critical and Doppler is therefore of considerable value. This is particularly true when the surgery involves arteriovenous malformations, vascular tumors, and arterial reconstruction. Although DCI is still new in the operating room, it has proven useful in a variety of surgical procedures, including those involving the brain, spine, liver, pancreas, kidneys, and cardiovascular system.

TECHNIQUE

With proper protection of the scanhead, most color-flow ultrasound scanners may be used for intraoperative applications. The size and shape of the transducer may limit its use for examination of some organs if surgical access is limited. Figure 9-1 shows a variety of conventional scanheads used with DCI systems for intraoperative scanning. Careful adherence to techniques of transducer preparation to ensure sterility is critical. Heat sterilization of transducers is impossible, and most transducers, particularly those with mechanical elements, are not suited for gas sterilization. It is therefore necessary to ensure sterility by enclosing the transducer in a sterile sheath. A variety of suitable plastic or latex sheaths for this purpose are commercially available. It is important that the sheath chosen for use fit the transducer head snugly, preventing redundant sheath material from interfering with scanhead contact. Before sheathing, the scanhead should be carefully cleansed with an antiseptic solution approved by the instrument manufacturer. Sterile gel is then applied to the scanhead and, with sterile precautions, the sheath is placed over the scanhead and its cable (Fig. 9-2A). Before use, the scanhead and its covering should be inspected to ensure that there are no defects in the covering that might compromise sterility.

Depending on the organ being scanned, acoustic contact is made by dripping sterile saline on the scanning site (Fig. 9-2B) or by partially filling the wound with sterile saline to provide a water path to the structure of interest. For examination of the liver and brain, scanning is usually performed directly on the organ, unless the abnormality is extremely superficial, in which case the standoff provided by a water path may be needed to avoid excessive near-field artifact.[3] For examination of the spinal cord, or of vessels after vascular repair, a water path is created by partially filling the operative field with sterile saline. When a water path is used, care should be taken to avoid agitating the saline solution used to fill the wound because the presence of gas bubbles in the solution interferes with flow imaging. Transducer frequencies of 5.0 to 7.5 MHz are generally used, depending on the application and the depth of the structure of interest.

INDICATIONS

Indications for intraoperative DCI include most of the established indications for intraoperative ultrasound imaging (Table 9-1). The addition of flow information provided by DCI is useful in almost all these applications and, in the case of arteriovenous malformations (AVMs) and following vascular repair, it is indispensable.

Central Nervous System

In the CNS, ultrasound imaging aids in the localization and characterization of subcor-

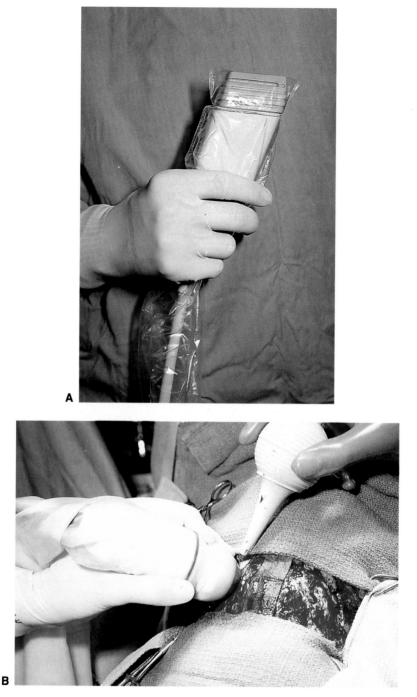

Fig. 9-2 Preparation for intraoperative scanning. **(A)** After cleaning, the transducer is enclosed in a sterile plastic sheath for intraoperative use. **(B)** Acoustical coupling is provided by irrigating the area to be examined with sterile saline or by partially filling the operative area with saline to create a water path.

Table 9-1 Indications for Intraoperative Ultrasonography

Brain and spine
  General
    Localization and characterization of subcortical lesions
    Identification of surgical complications
    Monitoring of resection
    Definition of cystic lesions
    Definition of extent of lesion
    Biopsy guidance
    Shunt placement
    Localization of foreign bodies and projectiles
    Localization of bone or disk fragments
    Shunting for hydrocephalus

  Arteriovenous malformation
    Localization
    Identification of nidus
    Identification of major feeding arteries and veins
    Selection of vessels for control
    Differentiation of AVM from hematoma
    Confirmation of complete resection
    Observation of hemodynamic changes during manipulation
    Evaluation of the effect of embolization
    Documentation of normal vessel flow

Abdomen
  Localization of cystic masses
  Identification of occult metastasis during hepatic resection
  Definition of the relationship of hepatic masses to major vessels before resection

Vascular
  Identification of sites for vessel clamping
  Identification of arteriovenous fistulas
  Localization of competent valve cusps
  Confirmation of adequacy of procedure and identification of residual disease
  Demonstration of technical defects after vascular repair
  Diagnosis of thrombosis

tical lesions, biopsy guidance, shunt placement, monitoring of resection, location of foreign bodies and projectiles, and identification of surgical complications. The intraoperative use of duplex and continuous-wave (CW) Doppler has also been reported to be useful in measuring blood flow, determining flow direction, and showing the hemodynamic effects of surgical maneuvers affecting AVMs.[4-6] In addition, Doppler has been used intraoperatively to monitor vasomotor reactivity to changes in CO_2 and to evaluate spinal cord circulation before and after treatment of spinal cord lesions. DCI is now being recognized as a useful adjunct to these recognized intraoperative applications and as an extension of conventional ultrasonographic imaging and Doppler methods.

Perhaps the most impressive contribution of DCI in neurosurgical procedures is in the real-time intraoperative assessment of AVMs. Typical brain and spinal cord AVMs are characterized by extensive vascularity with arteriovenous shunting and dilated afferent and efferent vessels. Because of the relatively high-flow states that characterize most AVMs of the CNS, these lesions and their associated vessels are readily imaged by DCI. The ability of DCI to image these lesions permits the surgeon to see the lesion and correctly evaluate its extent. This is particularly important for deeper portions of the lesion, where important vessels may be hidden from direct view. The correct identification of major vessels associated with an AVM is critical, because inadvertent ligation of a main draining vein before control of the arterial feeders to the lesion may result in catastrophic bleeding. Intraoperative angiography is a cumbersome means of monitoring AVM vasculature during resection. By showing the tangle of abnormal vessels characteristic of an AVM, DCI permits rapid differentiation of AVM from hematoma (Fig. 9-3).[7] Normal vessels are quickly differentiated from the abnormal vessels of the AVM, permitting rapid identification of the lesion, even if it is not visible from the surface. Flow within highly vascular lesions such as AVMs of the brain and spinal cord is demonstrated, aiding in localization and identification of major feeding arteries and

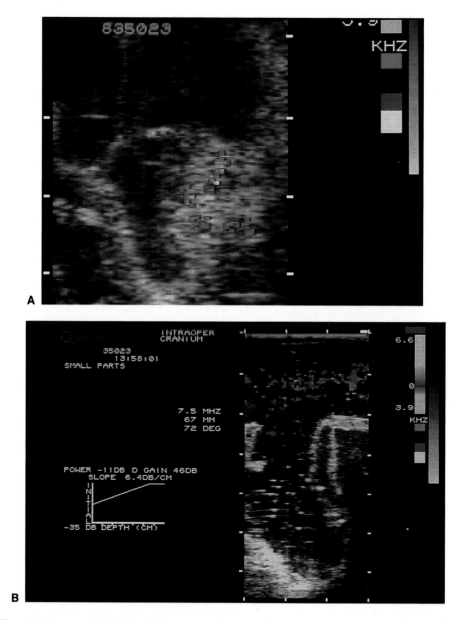

Fig. 9-3 Intracranial AVM. **(A)** Intraoperative scan shows increased vascularity associated with an intracerebral AVM. The AVM is clearly differentiated from the hypoechoic hematoma caused by bleeding from the lesion. **(B)** After evacuation of the hematoma and resection of the AVM, DCI shows only a fluid-filled cavity, with no residual flow in the area of the AVM. (From Merritt,[7] with permission.)

veins and in monitoring the effects of vessel ligation (Figs. 9-3 to 9-5). DCI aids in the selection of vessels for control and permits evaluation of the effects of embolization. Hemodynamic changes during manipulation may also be observed. Finally, DCI permits confirmation of completeness of resection. The usefulness of DCI in the surgical management of AVMs has been reported by several authors.[7-10] These studies confirm the value of intraoperative DCI for imaging cerebral and spinal AVMs as a useful adjunct in localizing vascular lesions, identifying feeding or draining vessels, and confirming intraoperative surgical excision. Rubin et al.[10] evaluated 12 patients who underwent AVM resection. Blood flow in the eight lesions was clearly evident, and major feeding arteries and draining veins, such as the superior sagittal sinus, were identified. DCI was used to differentiate adjacent hematoma from AVM in three patients, locate a small (6-mm) AVM deep in the brain in two patients, detect a deep major feeding artery in one patient, detect a residual unresected AVM in one patient, and confirm complete resection in all eight patients. In four patients DCI was judged to be of no use. In one patient the lesion was too deep for satisfactory flow imaging, in two patients technical factors interfered with imaging, and in the final patient the AVM was superficial and visual inspection was adequate, obviating any contribution of DCI. Our own experience with intracerebral and spinal AVMs confirms these observations.

Carotid and Peripheral Vessels

Arterial reconstruction may be complicated by vessel or graft occlusion, the formation of intimal flaps, and stenosis due to residual disease or technical defects. It is important that these complications be recognized and corrected as soon as possible to avoid the sequelae of embolization or thrombosis. Defects needing immediate repair are reported

to occur in 5 to 11 percent of patients undergoing endarterectomy.[11-13] In a series of 155 endarterectomies monitored by intraoperative real-time imaging, Flanigan et al.[14] identified technical defects in 43 vessels (28 percent). The most common defect was an intimal flap (73 percent of defects), followed by strictures (18 percent) and a variety of other problems including arterial kinks, residual plaque, and intraluminal thrombi (9 percent). Although intraoperative arteriography aids in the detection of these complications, it adds a small additional risk and is cumbersome to perform. As an alternative to angiography, Doppler ultrasound and real-time B-mode ultrasonic imaging are extremely useful techniques to monitor the technical success of reconstructive vascular operations.[11,12,15,16] When used at the time of carotid endarterectomy, intraoperative Doppler ultrasound may identify major defects requiring immediate repair, permitting immediate correction of significant technical problems, obviating the need for reoperation, and reducing the need for intraoperative arteriography. Doppler ultrasound is well accepted as a useful method for reducing operative complications in carotid endarterectomy. Initial reports of the value of intraoperative Doppler were based on the use of CW devices and spectral analysis alone. Zierler et al.[11] performed intraoperative arteriography in 150 consecutive endarterectomies and determined the contribution of pulsed spectral Doppler in 50 of these patients. Their ultrasound results agreed with their arteriography results with no false-negative results for sonography. Lack of improvement of the Doppler spectral changes after endarterectomy was found to be evidence of complications and was an indication for intraoperative angiography. Although useful, these nonimaging applications of Doppler require the performance of angiography to confirm and further characterize the abnormality responsible for the Doppler spectral abnormality. The addition of real-time imaging

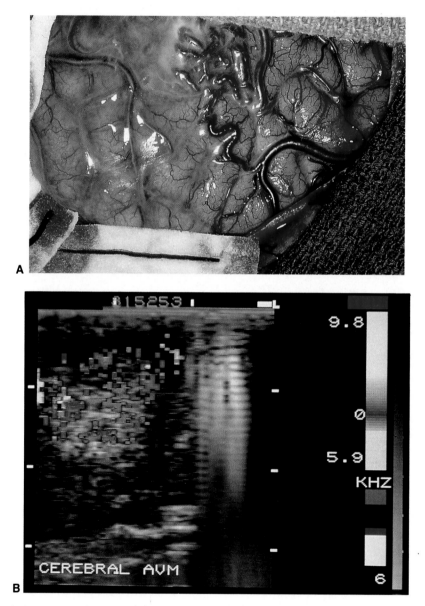

Fig. 9-4 Intracranial AVM. **(A)** Large vessels supplying a large intracerebral AVM are shown on the surface of the brain. **(B)** Intraoperative scan shows increased vascularity associated with the AVM. (*Figure continues.*)

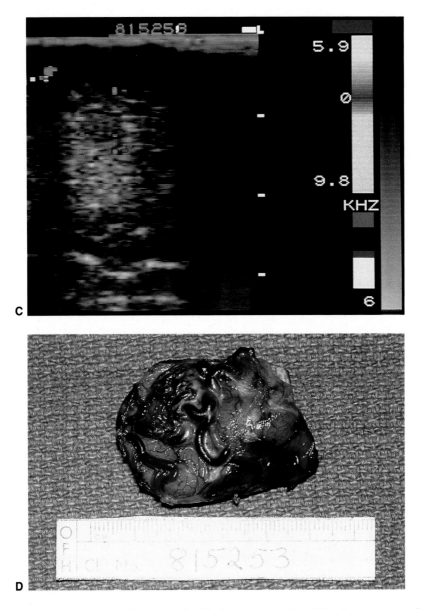

Fig. 9-4 (*Continued*). **(C)** After control of feeding vessels, the AVM shows no vascularity. **(D)** Resected lesion. (From Merritt,[8] with permission.)

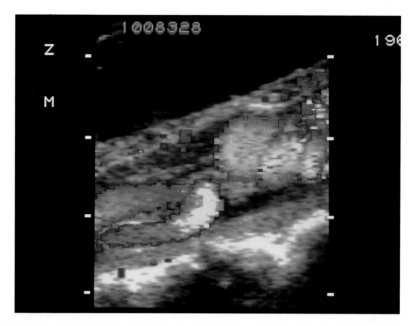

Fig. 9-5 Spinal cord AVM. A highly vascular AVM of the cervical spinal cord is shown. In this case intraoperative DCI was invaluable in identifying the main feeding vessels (left of image), helping the neurosurgeon obtain control over the blood supply to the lesion.

with the use of duplex equipment permits not only detection but also characterization of the nature of the complication.[14] Evidence of the value of intraoperative duplex carotid ultrasound after carotid artery reconstruction has been provided by Schwartz et al.[13] Intraoperative duplex imaging in 76 consecutive patients during 84 endarterectomies or carotid reconstruction procedures permitted identification of technical errors in 22 percent of patients and led to corrective measures during the surgical procedure in 11 percent. Among the findings with intraoperative sonography were residual stenosis, intraluminal thrombus, and loose debris. In this series, the authors concluded that surgical decision-making was affected by the use of intraoperative ultrasonography in a significant proportion of the patients studied.

DCI is a natural extension of duplex Doppler. Therefore it is not surprising that many of the benefits of DCI in evaluation of the peripheral arterial system apply in the intraoperative environment during arterial reconstructions. As in DCI examination of the peripheral arterial system, the ability of DCI to identify localized areas of stenosis and turbulence quickly with global Doppler sampling provided a significant advantage in the operative environment, where quick and accurate methods are particularly important. The techniques used for intraoperative vascular assessment are similar to those used in the examination of the peripheral arterial system, with the obvious additional requirement for sterile preparation of the transducer. In most cases, the ability to scan directly on the exposed vessel permits the use of high-frequency transducers (7.5 MHz or greater). Since most transducers have limited performance in the near field within the first centimeter or so of the transducer face, the use of a stand-off device or the creation of a

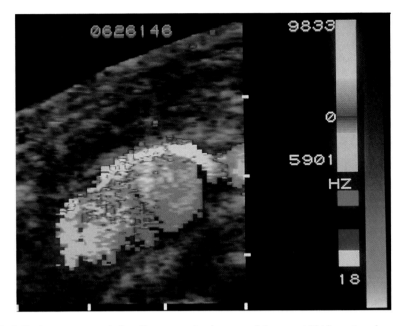

Fig. 9-6 Endarterectomy defect. Postoperative images of the carotid bifurcation show a high-velocity jet resulting from severe narrowing due to a large intimal flap that was not identified at the time of operation.

water path by filling the wound with sterile saline is generally necessary.

Although some surgeons have advocated routine use of intraoperative ultrasound to monitor arterial reconstruction, the availability of equipment may make this a difficult philosophy for most practices to implement, particularly if DCI instruments are required. In our practice, DCI is not used routinely but is readily available to assist the surgeon in difficult operative procedures. These include endarterectomy in patients with high stenoses or multiple areas of narrowing, in which the adequacy of the endarterectomy is difficult to assess, or patients in whom the reconstruction is found to be particularly difficult for other reasons.

Most of our experience has been in evaluation of the carotid artery at endarterectomy. Unrecognized surgical defects may result in restenosis or persistence of flow-restricting lesions that the surgery was performed to correct (Fig. 9-6). Intraoperative scanning may reduce these complications. Normal flow at the endarterectomy site is shown in Figure 9-7. The normal intraoperative appearance at the time of endarterectomy is that of a nonturbulent pattern of flow with a smooth vessel wall and no residual narrowing or evidence of high-velocity jets. At the site of the endarterectomy, small localized areas of flow separation and reversal are commonly noted, but in our experience these do not appear to be significant. Disturbed flow caused by residual plaque or wall irregularity is readily shown (Fig. 9-8). Small intimal flaps produce localized areas of turbulence that are readily recognized. Identification of such localized areas of flow disturbance permits spectral Doppler sampling to assess the hemodynamic significance of the defect. Peak systolic velocities of greater than 150

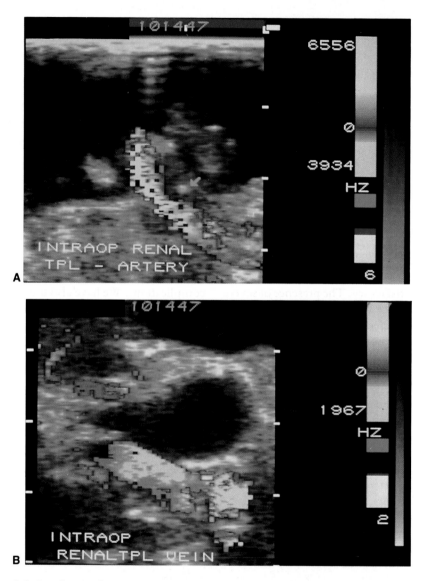

Fig. 9-9 Renal transplant. Intraoperative scans show **(A)** renal artery and **(B)** renal vein anastomoses to the iliac vessels. No significant narrowing or flow disturbance is seen.

operative ultrasound by providing global Doppler sampling, permitting the rapid identification of flow disturbances likely to affect surgical outcome. The finding of normal flow by DCI may be expected to provide a high degree of assurance that significant technical complications related to the operative procedure have been avoided, whereas the identification of flow disturbances permits immediate correction of the problem and reduces the need for reoperation and reduces delayed complications of thrombosis and restenosis. Early recognition of complications, reduction of operating time, less destruction of normal tissues, more precise surgery, and better operative results may all be promoted by the use of intraoperative ultrasonography. DCI is clearly a significant improvement of methods involving CW Doppler, pulsed spectral analysis, and duplex Doppler, in terms of ease of use and interpretation of results. Although DCI is currently in routine use in only a few centers, it is likely that demand for intraoperative DCI will steadily increase in coming years as its advantages and benefits become more widely known.

CRANIAL DOPPLER COLOR IMAGING

Pediatric Cranial Studies

The acoustic window provided by the open fontanels in infants permits the use of DCI in evaluation of normal and abnormal cerebral circulation.[21,22] Although normal intracranial vessels may be seen in great detail, few clinically useful applications of this capability have been reported. The sole exception is the noninvasive evaluation of intracerebral arteriovenous malformations. Recent duplex Doppler studies have identified alterations of cerebral blood flow associated with hydrocephalus and raise the possibility that expanded applications of cranial Doppler will emerge in the future.

EXAMINATION TECHNIQUE

DCI through the fontanels is performed by using techniques similar to those used to detect intracranial hemorrhage in neonates. Scanning through the anterior fontanel is performed in coronal, semiaxial, and parasagittal planes. Transducer frequencies of 5.0 to 7.5 MHz are used. Imaging is possible with both linear, curved linear, or phased array sector transducers. Scanning in an axial imaging plane through the posterior fontanel and the anterolateral fontanel or adjacent temporal squamosa is also possible in many infants, although lower imaging frequencies may be required to achieve adequate penetration.

NORMAL ANATOMY

Sagittal images through the anterior fontanel in the midline and angled laterally reveal the internal carotid arteries, the anterior cerebral arteries, and portions of the middle cerebral arteries. In the midline, each internal carotid artery may be visualized as it ascends adjacent to the sella. The anterior cerebral artery and the pericallosal and callosal marginal vessels are consistently demonstrated, along with cortical branches (Fig. 9-10). Flow in the internal cerebral veins as they accompany the posterior portions of the pericallosal arteries is also visible in this plane. The junction of the paired internal cerebral veins to form the vein of Galen just posterior to the splenium of the corpus callosum is visible, provided that an adequate Doppler angle can be achieved (Fig. 9-11).

Since the proximal portions of the middle cerebral arteries run essentially perpendicular to the sound beam, these vessels are not seen clearly. However, as the scan plane is directed more laterally, the opercular branches of the middle cerebral arteries become visible as they course within the sylvian fissure and anteriorly over the cortex. Coronal and semiaxial images obtained by angulation of the

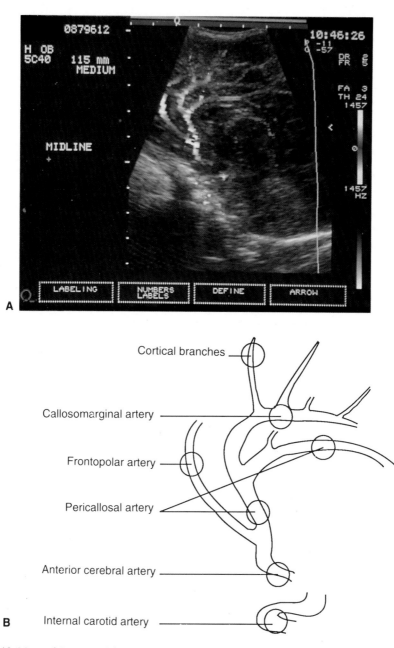

Fig. 9-10 Normal intracranial arteries—sagittal view. **(A)** Image through the anterior fontanel reveals the ICA, portions of the carotid siphon, and the anterior cerebral artery, including the pericallosal and callosal marginal branches. **(B)** The major vessels are identified.

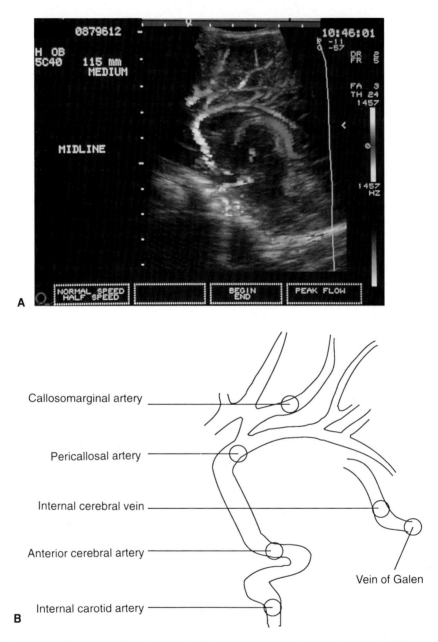

Fig. 9-11 Normal intracranial veins—sagittal view. **(A)** Image through the anterior fontanel reveals the internal cerebral vein (blue) as well as branches of the anterior cerebral artery. Note that the posterior portion of the pericallosal artery appears blue, similar to the vein, as a result of a change in its direction of flow relative to the transducer. **(B)** The major vessels are identified.

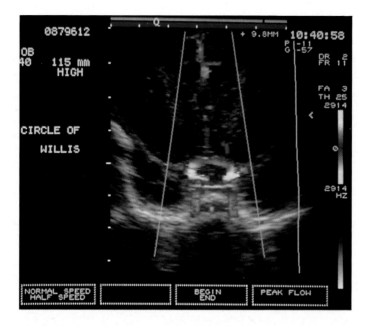

Fig. 9-12 Normal intracranial arteries—coronal view. Image through the anterior fontanel shows both ICAs adjacent to the sella and the proximal segments of both anterior cerebral arteries.

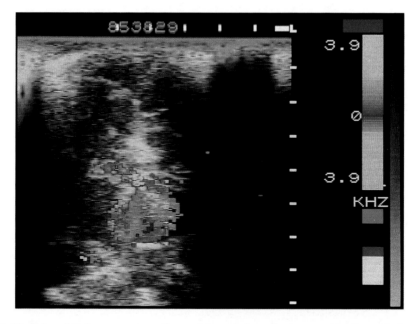

Fig. 9-13 Vein of Galen aneurysm. Coronal image through the anterior fontanel shows a large midline vascular mass with turbulent flow. Additional images showed major feeding vessels from the right posterior cerebellar artery. Angiography confirmed a large intracerebral AVM.

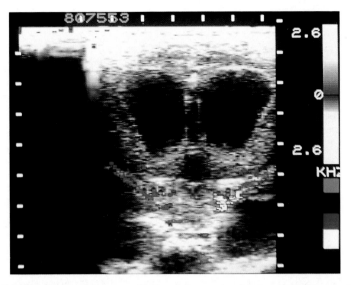

Fig. 9-14 ECMO. Coronal images of infant being maintained on ECMO reveal flow in the left ICA, but no flow in the right ICA. Flow is present in both middle cerebral arteries. The image was obtained at the time of peak systole in the left middle cerebral artery. Note the less saturated color in the right middle cerebral artery. This is due to a delay in filling of the right middle cerebral artery through collaterals. Hydrocephalus is present.

transducer posteriorly in the anterior fontanel allow visualization of the circle of Willis and the anterior and middle cerebral arteries (Fig. 9-12).

Several studies[21-23] have documented the efficacy of DCI in providing detailed imaging of intracranial vasculature. Wong et al.[22] examined 14 neonates via the anterior fontanel and, whenever possible, with views through the posterior fontanel and temporal bone. The anterior cerebral, M1 segment of the middle cerebral artery, distal internal carotid artery (ICA), and basilar artery were demonstrated consistently. Portions of the vertebral, distal middle cerebral artery and the posterior cerebral artery were frequently visualized. The anterior fontanel approach was shown to be the most useful in identifying most of the major intracranial arteries and veins by DCI. Mitchell et al.[21] used DCI to scan 53 healthy full-term infants within 3 days of birth and were able to image the basilar artery, anterior and middle cerebral arteries, and ICA in all infants. The vertebral, posterior cerebral, superior cerebellar, and posterior communicating arteries were seen in most infants. A pitfall involving imaging of the distal portion of the ICA was noted: this vessel could be confused with the proximal portion of the anterior cerebral artery or cavernous sinus if real-time images were not interpreted carefully. These investigators also reported variant patterns of flow including tortuous basilar arteries, reversed flow in the posterior communicating artery, and inferior angulation of the proximal portions of the anterior cerebral arteries.

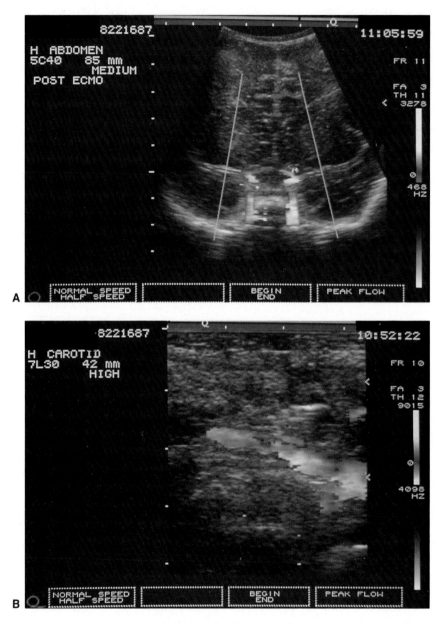

Fig. 9-15 CCA reanastomosis after ECMO. **(A)** Coronal images of intracranial vessels 1 week following ECMO and reanastomosis of the right CCA reveal normal and symmetric flow. **(B)** Longitudinal view of the right CCA at the anastomotic site reveals good flow with no narrowing or significant flow disturbance.

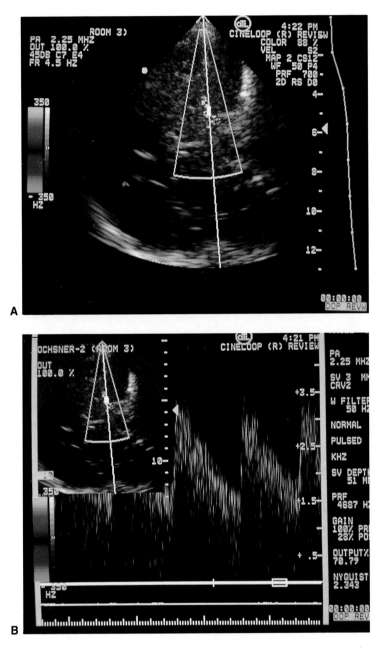

Fig. 9-16 Transcranial DCI. DCI now permits imaging of intracranial vessels in adults as well as infants and is being investigated as an adjunct to conventional transcranial Doppler. **(A)** Axial image through the temporal bone shows a portion of the left middle cerebral artery. **(B)** The Doppler waveform is normal.

ABNORMALITIES OF CRANIAL FLOW

The conditions most extensively evaluated by DCI include AVMs and aneurysms of the vein of Galen and changes in cerebral blood flow in infants undergoing extracorporeal membrane oxygenation (ECMO). Tessler et al.[24] have reported excellent correlation of DCI and angiography findings in five infants with cerebral AVMs. Arterial feeders and major draining veins were visualized in all five patients. In three patients with aneurysms of the vein of Galen, sonography showed a cystic structure with rapid or swirling flow (Fig. 9-13). DCI may also be helpful in evaluating the effect of embolic or operative therapy in infants with AVMs.[24,25] DCI has also been reported to aid in the diagnosis of intracerebral AVMs in adults as well as infants. Becker et al.[26] evaluated two patients with proven AVMs and were able to identify the major afferent feeding vessels and the venous drainage in both patients.

ECMO is an increasingly common procedure used to treat infants with severe and potentially reversible pulmonary impairment. To perform this procedure, a membrane oxygenator is used with arterial access through the common carotid artery (CCA). At completion of the procedure the CCA is often ligated. The effects of CCA ligation on intracerebral circulation have been studied by using DCI (Fig. 9-14).[22,27,28] Wong et al.[22] examined 10 neonates who had undergone ECMO. In this group of patients, DCI demonstrated occlusion of the right ICA and reversal of flow through the ipsilateral A1 segment. Increased flow on the contralateral side and in the basilar artery was observed in several patients. Mitchell et al.[28] have used DCI to evaluate collateral flow patterns after CCA ligation in 58 infants. Using criteria based on the direction of flow in the right ICA at sites proximal and distal to the right posterior communicating artery, three flow patterns were described. Anterior communicating artery dominance, with retrograde flow in the entire right ICA, was common during ECMO but did not persist. Posterior communicating artery dominance, with antegrade right ICA flow distal to the right posterior communicating artery, was common shortly after ECMO and later. External carotid artery dominance ($N = 16$), with antegrade flow throughout the right ICA, was noted in 53 percent of studies more than 1 month after ECMO but in only 9 percent of earlier studies. We have also used DCI to evaluate the CCA after reanastomosis following ECMO, documenting normal flow in most cases (Fig. 9-15).[29]

Transcranial Doppler

A final potential area of application of cranial DCI is for transcranial examinations in adults (Fig. 9-16). DCI is currently being evaluated as an adjunct to conventional transcranial Doppler. Although its efficacy has not been established, DCI may enhance the identification of intracranial vessels for Doppler sampling.

Summary

In infants normal intracranial vessels may be seen in detail by using DCI. This capability is most useful in the initial or follow-up examination of infants with intracerebral AVMs. Aside from this, few clinically important applications of DCI to image the intracranial vessels have been reported.

REFERENCES

1. Merritt CRB, Coulon R, Connolly E: Intraoperative neurosurgical ultrasound: transdural and transfontanelle applications. Radiology 148:513, 1983
2. Machi J, Sigel B, Kurohiji T, et al: Operative ultrasound guidance for various surgical procedures. Ultrasound Med Biol 16:37, 1990
3. Merritt CRB, Voorhies RM, Connolly E,

Coulon R: Intraoperative neurosurgical ultrasound. Semin Ultrasound CT MR 6:31, 1985

4. Giller CA, Finn SS: Intraoperative measurement of spinal cord blood velocity using pulsed Doppler ultrasound. A case report. Surg Neurol 32:387, 1989

5. Giller CA, Meyer YJ, Batjer HH: Hemodynamic assessment of the spinal cord arteriovenous malformation with intraoperative microvascular Doppler ultrasound: case report. Neurosurgery 25:270, 1989

6. Hassler W, Thron A, Grote EH: Hemodynamics of spinal dural arteriovenous fistulas. An intraoperative study. J Neurosurg 70:360, 1989

7. Merritt CRB: Doppler color flow imaging: J Clin Ultrasound 15:591, 1987

8. Merritt CRB: Real-time Doppler color flow imaging: other applications. p. 42. In Bernstein EF (ed): Recent Advances in Noninvasive Diagnostic Techniques in Vascular Disease. CV Mosby, St. Louis, 1990

9. Black KL, Rubin JM, Chandler WF, McGillicuddy JE: Intraoperative color-flow Doppler imaging of AVM's and aneurysms. J Neurosurg 68:635, 1988

10. Rubin JM, Hatfield MK, Chandler WF, et al: Intracerebral arteriovenous malformations: intraoperative color Doppler flow imaging. Radiology 170:219, 1989

11. Zierler RE, Bandyk DF, Thiele BL: Intraoperative assessment of carotid endarterectomy. J Vasc Surg 1:73, 1984

12. Bandyk DF, Zierler RE, Thiele BL: Detection of technical error during arterial surgery by pulsed Doppler spectral analysis. Arch Surg 119:421, 1984

13. Schwartz RA, Peterson GJ, Noland KA, et al: Intraoperative duplex scanning after carotid artery reconstruction: a valuable tool. J Vasc Surg 7:620, 1988

14. Flanigan DP, Douglas DJ, Machi J, et al: Intraoperative ultrasonic imaging of the carotid artery during carotid endarterectomy. Surgery 100:893, 1986

15. Barnes RW: Intraoperative monitoring in vascular surgery. Ultrasound Med Biol 12:919, 1986

16. Barnes RW, Nix ML, Wingo JP, Nichols BT: Recurrent *versus* residual carotid stenosis. *Incidence detected by Doppler ultrasound.* Ann Surg 203:652, 1986

17. Beard JD, Scott DJA, Skidmore R, et al: Operative assessment of femorodistal bypass grafts using a new Doppler flowmeter. Br J Surg 76:925, 1989

18. Okuhn SP, Stoney RJ: Intraoperative use of ultrasound in arterial surgery. Surg Clin North Am 70:61, 1990

19. Bandyk DF, Jorgensen RA, Towne JB: Intraoperative assessment of in situ saphenous vein arterial grafts using pulsed Doppler spectral analysis. Arch Surg 121:292, 1986

20. Spencer TD, Goldman MH, Hyslop JW, et al: Intraoperative assessment of in situ saphenous vein bypass grafts with continuous-wave Doppler probe. Surgery 96:874, 1984

21. Mitchell DG, Merton DA, Mirsky PJ, Needleman L: Circle of Willis in newborns: color Doppler imaging of 53 healthy full-term infants. Radiology 172:201, 1989

22. Wong WS, Tsuruda JS, Liberman RL, et al: Color Doppler imaging of intracranial vessels in the neonate. AJR 152:1065, 1989

23. Mitchell DG, Merton D, Needleman L, et al: Neonatal brain: color Doppler imaging. I. Technique and vascular anatomy. Radiology 167:303, 1988

24. Tessler FN, Dion J, Viñuela F, et al: Cranial arteriovenous malformations in neonates: color Doppler imaging with angiographic correlation. AJR 153:1027, 1989

25. Ciricillo SF, Schmidt KG, Silverman NH, et al: Serial ultrasonographic evaluation of neonatal vein of Galen malformations to assess the efficacy of interventional neuroradiological procedures. Neurosurgery 27:544, 1990

26. Becker GM, Winkler J, Hoffmann E, Bogdahn U: Imaging of cerebral arteriovenous malformations by transcranial colour-coded real-time sonography. Neuroradiology 32:280, 1990

27. Mitchell DG, Merton D, Desai H, et al: Neonatal brain: color Doppler imaging. II. Altered flow patterns from extracorporeal membrane oxygenation. Radiology 167:307, 1988

28. Mitchell DG, Merton DA, Graziani LJ, et al: Right carotid artery ligation in neonates: classification of collateral flow with color Doppler imaging. Radiology 175:117, 1990

29. Adolph V, Bonis S, Falterman K, Arensman R: Carotid artery repair after pediatric extracorporeal membrane oxygenation. J Pediatr Surg 25:867, 1990

Index

Page numbers followed by f refer to figures; those followed by t refer to tables.